AATMA YOGA

DECODE THE SECRETS WITHIN AND REJUVENATE YOURSELF

KORAK DAY

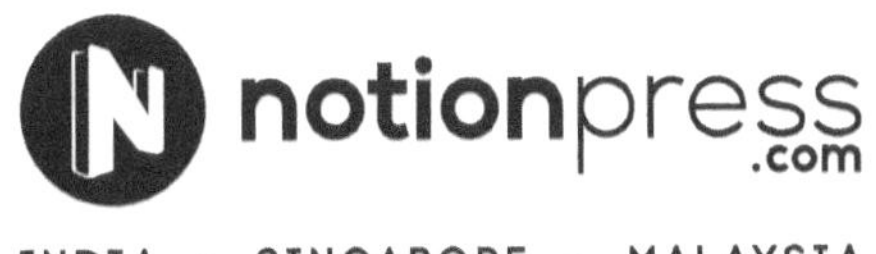

Notion Press

Old No. 38, New No. 6
McNichols Road, Chetpet
Chennai - 600 031

First Published by Notion Press 2019

ISBN 978-1-64587-540-6

Dedicated to

All those people ever born on the earth, who lived their whole life as humane. Not those who showed off being humane, but those whose actions were immaculately humane.

CONTENTS

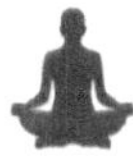

ACKNOWLEDGMENT

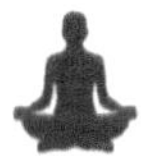

A published book is not just the contribution of the writer, I believe. So many take part in bringing it to the final version.

Dr. Dipak N Patel of USA is always the first one to thank for my Art creations, just like Theo van Gogh, the brother of one of the most celebrated artist (painter) Vincent van Gogh. Dipak's unfailing financial support allowed Korak Day to devote himself entirely to his creations of art and the works for serving humanity with selfless love.

Korak went for a week to write his one fiction and one nonfiction books in solitude to the Himalayas. There he stayed in Afia Homestay in Lepchajagat, Darjeeling. The owners Anil Tamang, his sweet wife Monika Tamang and little daughter Afia were such generous hosts. They encouraged him to write (as he was alone here) and supported him during his misfortunes at his Ashram back in Kolkata. They also took out to make him feel happy as he was sad. One of the unwanted child Korak has adopted since 2004 broke his upper arm and also they had a road accident where they were unhurt while others died. Anil and Monika even did not take any lodging and fooding charges from him, saying, "who takes money from their elder brother?"

Taking out time to create, along with all his humanitarian works that Korak does these days, would have been impossible. But there are a few people whose infinitely large selfless hearts only could make him have time and energy to create.

First two are Gopal Day and Chandragupt Day, Korak's first two Satwik Shishyays who are selflessly taking care of every problem and constraint that he faces. Gopal Day was born an Avatar whom you cannot see with Kaliyugi eyes, and the other is born Md Afzal, who is physically there. There is a third person named Koyel or

Krishna Chakraborty, who was sent to me by my daughter Goddess Durga. These are the matters of Soul Aatma and for the one who has realized Aatma Yoga, can only decode this.

I cannot finish this book without mentioning Renuka MD from my publisher's company, who always inspired me to write. She helped me in all possible ways under her capacity so that I could publish and take my books to the world.

PROLOGUE

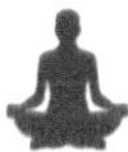

Money – Food – Shelter – Luxury, you have them all but isn't it frustrating to become depressed, often? Are you longing for something that will make you real 'happy'?

Aatma Yoga is your custom-made solution.

I am not writing this book for everyone, as I cannot, and I am aware of that. But, it would be an excellent idea to reach most people, though! We all have a soul within, but as we are busy with our body and mind, we tend to ignore our Soul. At present, I am only writing for those who seek a better life. Your life would be better off by solving a followings struggle/issue you are dealing with, now:

i. Improved relationships,

ii. Health-wealthy life,

iii. Worry-free tomorrow,

iv. Well-defended priorities,

v. Permanent peace,

vi. Free from any color of slavery,

vii. Non-ending joy,

viii. Having monetary satisfaction,

ix. Acknowledge their unique brilliance within,

x. The fulfillment of their inner potentials,

xi. Maintained happiness,

xii. Being a role model.

If you are struggling with even one of them, then this book is yours to rejuvenate your remaining life, to the fullest.

This book is also created for those 'people' in your life, who are longing to be closer to you. Also, for those who are part of your life. Your friends, family, relative, customers, audience, fans, etc.

No, it is not a marketing tactic, it is a necessity!

'We' are not 'me.' We can never make things better for us if we do not co-exist with people surrounding us. It must also be easier to make that bridge for those people you get in touch with ever, in life. If there isn't a bridge between that person and you, then life becomes difficult. All the bad things follow freely then!

We 'have to' leave being 'me' and get into the 'we' mode and then it takes two to tango. That other person who would like to deal with you needs to make the bridge with you. Also for you to make a bridge or even to help them make the bridge on which both of you need to walk and share.

Now you know why it would be so crucial for both you and those who you are close to or want to be close to, to have this book? Let us work together in making the world a beautiful, joyful, and peaceful place for you and your universe.

Chapter 1

A STORY FOR YOU

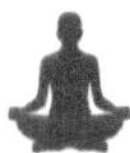

A tiny disclaimer: this book is for those who are adults. Cultures and laws they say come and goes. Many would moot for the age of being an adult. So you decide for yourself, at what age you are an adult; eighteen or puberty?

I meanwhile would go with nature.

At the end of each day, it's your personal Joy and personal Peace within; that's all that matters. If you are fine, then the whole world around you seems bright to you. And if you suffer, no one cares! Well, friends and families would care for some days till when you are no more or down. But after sometimes we all get used to any kind of loss. Don't we all move on?

It is "you" that must matter to you, primarily! Let us do good to ourselves now, and when we are beautiful, we will take care of others too.

The movement of the Earth does not change in its speed/direction if its inhabitants go through hell. That brings about no change anywhere. The sun too does the same routine of the so-called rising in the east and setting in the west. It never stops bringing light, heat, and warmth to its inhabitants. We alone, have to go through our own shit!

So Let there be Light.

Rose was late to wake up today. She has a hangover from yesterday's party, late at night. The daylight peeped through the window curtains. She felt heaviness on her breast, she shifted herself to find it was a hairy tanned hand. She held it and removed it away while getting up in haste.

She didn't know the nude man lying on her side with a substantial early morning erection on. Seeing her clothes lying all over the floor, she started to shake the man to wake him up. She didn't care to notice his curling brown hair falling on his handsome white face. Rose tucked her light blond hair behind her ear. With anger and disgust in her eyes, gave a strong push to the man, she didn't know who he was.

Deep blue eyes guarded by lush dark eyelashes widened with wonder and turned into anger. "Where am I, how am I here?"

The man didn't reply and got up from the bed and was looking for his clothes. Rose was furious, she jumped out of bed and jumped at the tall man and pulled his hair. He turned back and gave a tight slap to her. Still, she didn't leave his hair.

"How I am here, tell me, now!"

He gives a punch on her face, and it starts to bleed. "You sexy bitch! Get off me!"

Rose fell to a side of the bed but stood back and rushed to the man with a vengeance. The man now was furious, he came forward to her and held her arms to her back. Her breast bounces on his face, and he had a cunning smile.

"Why are you doing this at all! We had a nice time here, finished, now pack up!"

"You had a nice time!"

"You too, bitch, err sexy bitch" he plays with her breasts with his face.

"Let me go, but how I came here?" She was trying hard to release herself from his grip.

"You drunk a lot, danced a lot and then when the party finished, you couldn't open the door of your car. Thank me I was around and brought you in my car to my home. Where to take you? It was you who were falling all over me."

"Thanks, let me go know."

"Go, no," he makes her fall on her back on the bed and jumped on her, kissing her.

"Stop it, I have to go, I have an urgent meeting!"

"I will not let you go before repeating the pleasures of the night!" Tired and exhausted, she mustered all her strength and tried to punch him. He was fast to save his face.

"Is that the way you say thank you?" He forces himself into her, and Rose screams, "use a rubber, I am on periods."

"You are welcome!" and he laughs.

Beverly Hills, Rodeo Drive seemed crowded to Rose, as she was driving in her car back home.

She has a swollen lip, and a bruised nose, and her green eyes looked dark with dark eye bags. She was looking at her face on the rearview mirror in front of her. She puts on her huge dark shades and a scarf on her face to hide the bruises. Now she looked calm, again.

As she drives down the block, tears drop from behind her dark glasses. She lifts her head to a side and sees the Museum of Tolerance.

She parks her car at a side. She looks at the sand-colored building of the Museum designed as steps to walk upon, and reach to the sky maybe, she thought.

Looking at the Museum of Tolerance, she remembered how in 1994, she came here as a teenager. Her mother and her present husband were with her too. She was curious to visit Anne Frank's room in the Secret Annex. Then how her mother left, and while she was alone going through the diary pages of Anne, she met her husband to be. It was love at first sight, courtesy Anne. Everything looked promising and dreamlike.

The life they say is harsh, and that's why we all love to dream and imagine beautiful things. How, as a teenager, you had imaginations and hopes for a beautiful life with a loving life-partner! Children, a dream job and a house in luxury. All looks so hopeful and rosy!

Even if your name is Rose yourself, but to Shakespeare's, 'what's in a name,' I add my nonfiction. 'What's in a name, a soul by any name has to go through the rape of the emotions of life.' Obviously, who likes rape, no one likes it! What to do, we have to learn to spread our legs wide and lol, enjoy!

Do you know we become unaware that we also have options to either stop the rapist or even rape the rapist back? Rose too, was spreading her legs wide and 'existing' with the various rapists of her spirits and dreams. And now even her body!

Her parents never had time for her, except whatever money could buy. She felt she needed, something different from them. Within a couple of years of marriage, things halted. Husband had less time for her and more time for his business and sexcapades.

Her firstborn died due to SIDS, Sudden Infant Death Syndrome.

After the divorce with her dream husband she met at the Museum of Tolerance, she had a bumpy five years. She married three times and had thirteen serious boyfriends, but no one gave her what she craved for. But she never had put them in points, what she sought.

The situation at her job was worse!

Looking at the museum building, she realized that all she got in her job was stagnancy, no steps above. She felt her bosses could never harness her talents. She changed jobs often, as often as her boyfriends.

Lately, she started her own business, leaving her high paying job. She was a script manager at a famous Screenwriter's Agent in Santa Monica Blvd in Beverly Hills.

She works now alone on her business from her home, but she feels her business is not growing. Since the last sixteen months, she never dated anymore or had a quickie even.

She longed for something, someone, but she couldn't put her fingers on those. This was her first sex after sixteen months. She hated men for their chauvinistic nature, and she was sure all men were evil. She neither stopped the rapist, not rape the rapist back.

The tissue box was empty as she took out the last sheet to wipe her non-stop tear shower. A man with black eyes, black hair and a light brown skin tone approached her car.

"I am a YouTube Vlogger SoulDost, a dost is a friend in Indian. Can I ask you, what do you know about India."

Wiping her tears, "Nothing, and I don't care."

"Why not, India has all the answers, especially for those that melts and flows from your beautiful eyes. Try Aatma Yoga there."

Chapter 2

MODERN PROBLEMS

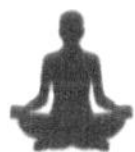

What is the point looking at the problems that 'me,' 'we,' 'us' go through, with a magnifying glass? The light within is dim without knowing the darkest evil, the rapist of our spirits. Come let's remember it thoroughly and then take the steps to a permanent brilliance, within 'me,' 'we' and 'us.'

Please tick those that are your problems too, that you want to overcome.

☐ Must we skip the money situation or take it upfront? Debts, EMI, upcoming festivals, feasts, parties et all, no money, no security, no nothing. How much money can give you financial security? If you earn 7500, you think a 10k would be better, and upon 10k a 15 seems unavoidable. The madness of the matrix of money.

☐ Self Esteem is so crucial, and a lack of it is bitter. Endless issues with it and the distractions always keep on knocking the door. Self-confidence keeps fluctuating these days.

☐ As I mentioned earlier, we are never happy being 'me.' We all crave and pursue lasting relationships. Loneliness is closest to all the unhappiness and then, we would do anything to avoid that.

☐ A massive problem for a modern man these days is to have the winner's mindset. The mindset required for personal development is proportional to the desired personal growth. We all strive to develop a limitless mindset. So that life continues to flow therein without a hindrance.

☐ The most significant wealth of life is our health and that of our family members. Without health or handicapped health, we get the most significant constraint in daily life.

- ☐ Happiness is what everyone seeks, but everyone ill-treats the source. Whenever we are in short supply of the happiness factor, we get into depressions and the similar.

- ☐ When our priorities are not well defined or clarified, we make our own and that of our loved one's life, boring. We are useless when we do not know our priorities, or they are not well defined. Lack of well-defended priorities in life is a significant cause of fights. Also, for the secret wars amongst family/colleagues/acquaintances.

- ☐ How often do we seek troubled-times and enjoy them? A permanent peace within or a lack of it causes anxieties. This leads to further peace-hijacks in the family or office.

- ☐ All kinds of issues and problems that our children or our spouses go through lead to the enormous challenges we face. Many parents put everything with their children's or spouse's life, and a small mismatch is lethal.

- ☐ For financial security, we often get engrossed in taking up a job/work that we are not passionate about. Thus we skip our inner potentials, and they, in return, makes us skip peace.

- ☐ If not the world around us, but we know our negativity. But being positive in quite uncool in your surroundings often. And that becomes a massive problem for you within.

- ☐ Like Rose, it is a massive problem for a modern person to get the real job they know they will be happy with. An office with understanding and cooperating colleagues becomes another associated problem. We often get inspired to leave a position to start our own business. But often the decision dilutes after failures or hardships. Then begins the turmoils within.

- ☐ For many women, it is a huge problem to deal with their chauvinistic husband or partners.

- ☐ Many people go through various forms of slavery given to them. Their family members, society, etc. provide them with slavery. They want to do something good, but due to enslavement, they are not able to.

☐ Religion and the related slavery is often a source for problems for followers. The dictates make the life of its followers as prisoners, unbearable, and hellish.

☐ What will happen tomorrow is a colossal tension amongst people. Wondering about tomorrow and losing peace on it is also a huge problem.

☐ There is also a spiritual problem amongst thoughtful and well-read people. Here we want to be the role model or a celebrity or a hero or heroine whom people look up to, or they want to look up upon. That is the cause of a lot of overacting and overreaction, which often is unnecessary.

Besides these above problems which are global, there are many local problems too. Some could be quite funny when mentioned and quite dangerous too if left from this compilation. When I did my survey for this book, I found people generally have these problems also:

☐ Waking up in early morning and getting prepared for office.

☐ Attending long duration lectures for a subject in college/ institutes of their dislike.

☐ After getting a degree or a diploma, still, we are unsure where to go.

☐ Dipping a biscuit in the tea and losing half or more, in it.

☐ Public places that remain dirty, and the local government sleeps over it.

☐ Lack of security related issue with women and gays.

☐ Internet stopped or disconnected when you are ordering something important. Or an online offer that would be off soon.

☐ Buying you last minute Tatkal ticket online and the internet becomes snail speed. Then you discover no seats available, that day.

☐ Forgetting to visit the toilet before sleep. Then removing huge blankets in the night and coming out of the bed, in the winters, to pee.

☐ When your birthday falls in the month end.

- ☐ Paying more money than required. You are not carrying change, and the ticket checker tells you to bring change. When you have even a little less change, it's pandemonium. Then the moral lectures on poor people cheated of the money they worked so hard for.

- ☐ The ever increasing and unmanaged pollutions.

- ☐ Lack of toilets in public places.

- ☐ Spent your pocket money for the month, in the first week.

- ☐ You want to charge your phone while in bed, and the charging point is far.

- ☐ Lack of toilets in public transports going to some far off places.

- ☐ Forgot something important while buying your grocery. Now neither you could go back, nor you could do without.

- ☐ You were busy somewhere, and you lost count of the whistles in the pressure cooker.

- ☐ Waking up early morning after a late night sleep.

- ☐ Going to the office, especially when for them their office/work sucks!

- ☐ Going through the traffic is another major problem, while we create one.

- ☐ Reaching office/work-place late and the consequences faced on being late.

- ☐ Trying to get a leave for some urgent work, from your grumpy HR.

- ☐ Neighbors throwing their trash in front of your house.

- ☐ Strange and loud ring tones in public places.

- ☐ When you are in a new or foreign city and end up paying five times more.

- ☐ Uncleaned and overflowing sewage.

- ☐ Overfilled and spilling public trash bins.

☐ Overcrowded public transports.

☐ No tickets are available to book due to lack of trains and overcrowded local trains, but unlimited budgets for bullet trains.

☐ You pay a considerable amount to get a train ticket in Premium Tatkal. But a train ticket checker does not mind overcrowding the reserved compartments.

☐ Pickpockets in public places.

☐ Tangled earphones and untangling them.

☐ Loudspeakers.

There are many many more similar problems that we all go through these times, but I would stop here. Thank God, I did.

Chapter 3

SOLUTIONS:
POPULAR VS. REAL

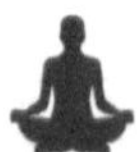

REALITY

Jamshid (name changed), "But why don't you understand, I can't pay you so many US$, I am left with one kidney now! I sold the other one to flee Iran to save prosecution because of what Allah made me, a Gay! Don't I have a right to have a hope to live in peace? (sigh) And I thought America is the land of freedom."

Rose was very strict in her business. She never gives up on her own established ethics in running her business. "You have to spend a $4997 to have a decent event arranged for your musical night with Kam... whatever."

"It's a Kamancheh. Do you realize how important it is for me, this performance."

"Everything is important for everyone so is my business for me. Jamshid, I am not doing charity, so let's not waste both our times here."

"Rose, I have $3500 that I saved working so hard in Canada, an alien land. Stayed alone with no friends so that one day I could come and mesmerize LA. With my musical talent, and that would be the beginning of peace and joy, I was craving as a child in Iran."

"Forget peace and joy in LA; moreover, you are a vagabond, running from everywhere."

"Do you know the life of an Allah-created-woman in a man's body, in that Allah following Iran? How much do you know about the problems of the rest of the world? But I see now that America is no different than the rest of the world. There it's the atrocities of the God damning Government-slavery. And here it's the God damning money-slavery."

REAL

Well, now we have the devil in our hands. We know our needs, wishes, desires, to do list, missions, etc. All this exists to keep us away from the real thing. This real thing is what all human souls seek. That which hides within us. But that needs decoding to be deciphered!

This is the destination of this book and that we will get enlightened with.

Let us find out what are the solutions we had been getting from the solution-givers of modern humans, all these years.

All we got from them in every possible color, shape, name, variety are nothing but a lot and lots of "words." We can muster all the words and master all the thoughts. But if we cannot apply that with the satisfaction-nod coming from within, what's the use for them? That is the reason why all these 'word' that comes from outside of us fails. We meed the solutions to come from within period.

Let's for a change, come back to our beloved Rose.

Rose kept working with her business but kept recalling the message from the YouTuber.

She tried hard to remember the message, but she couldn't! She remembered that she has a CarMemo App installed on her car. That records through AllView Camera everything that happens in and around the vehicle.

She arrives in her office-home to a lot of messages on her answering machine. The messages keep talking, but she vanishes in her thoughts. She is taking her shower, and she decides to check something on her latest iPhone.

"Why not, India has all the answers, especially for those that melts and flows from your beautiful eyes. Try Aatma Yoga there."

Rose has twinkles in her eyes, and a smile breaks out from her tensed and worried face. She goes back to the shower, and she puts her fingers over her face. Water spills from the gaps of the fingers on her face, and she is all full of smile.

She leaves the shower and puts on her shower gown, drying her hair. She goes to her MacBook Pro, opens it, searches about India. She looks with hope, wonder, and anticipation.

POPULAR

Starting at the nonfiction again, we will now have the solutions we generally get to take care of our modern problems. There are many groups, individuals and people with various options of sure-solutions which sure-fails.

Without any judgment, I will state them to you here. The net is full of them, but I present a glimpse. There are following networks that work as "popular sure-solutions" these days:

i. Religious Networks

Endless religions, sects, gurus, priestly-sermons, Friday-lectures are a party to that. The authority of books, buildings and the brigades of the so-called powerful-authorities too. You do not have the option to deny them. Cannot dismiss them without their fear-induced scare-offs. Even evil murders on denial, in the name of their version of divinity.

ii. The Medical Network

Like the religious network, this too is a vast network. With a massive spread of its web across the society, everywhere. These people come with their own set of authorities. This is directly proportional to 'do what I order you' or be damned. From psychiatrists to doctors to medical journals to pharmaceutical companies, unavoidable.

iii. The Media Network

The contents of the magazine, newspaper, television, cinema are programmed by the rich. They have a network working for an ulterior motive or a set of objectives. They too try all under their capacity to solve the modern-day problems. Do they solve them or fuel them, is not my work to tell.

iv. The Tamed-Elephant Network

Sir Gorge Bernard Shaw in 'Man and Superman' talked about using the tamed elephants to catch the wild ones. They are secretly planted (voluntarily or even involuntarily) amongst the society, around us. They are like vultures looking around to catch their prey: the humble, meek and the sad.

v. The Blind Network

Often, the blinds lead the blinds to their own darkness, no less. How frequently you would meet such people who would be such an earful? Then they secretly mislead you with the most sugar-coated toppings and talking.

vi. The Celebrity Network

Celebrities in various fields, in place of doing their job, would become false-leaders. They act as leaders of the souls of people with their motivated and misleading comments. You sure must have known their scams of accepting substantial benefits in return of their' opinions.'

vii. The Wannabe Superpower Networks

Big countries around your country or some faraway country who wants to be a superpower. They spend a lot of money and privileges to the greedy public figures of the country they wish to dominate. Thus creating soft enemies amongst countrymen. There are many examples you will find in your own state of such people.

Be aware of looking around before you take the next step while doing your daily chores. This leads to the next part: what 'must' be the solution, then?

HIDDEN SOLUTIONS

The solution that most of the people in our modern times are seeking is not there outside of us. It's not like taking a chill pill, and you get chilled out! Popular solution these days are like you have a headache and take an aspirin. But does that solve a problem, or do they make you numb to the challenge?

We who practice Aatma Yoga, we delve deep into the cause of the headache first. Then we get the treatment done to rectify the pin-pointed cause.

Making actions on reactions is futile and is a business strategy. Making good-actions on the bad-actions stops the wrong steps.

All the solutions you need for your best are all programmed within you, already at birth.

No outsider with any degree of authority could ever solve your problem at the best of your need. Well, they could, at the most, try to, but they mostly fail or succeed partially or temporarily! 'Introspection,' or getting to know yourself is the first successful step. This is true for any man, woman, or a transgender person, located anywhere on Earth.

Once you take the first step successfully, you don't need any external guide, book, pope, imam, pandit, or a guru to solve any of your needs or drawbacks! Post that first step, all you would ever need will speak from within and guide you best with your own uniqueness.

We all, each one of us, is unique!

Please don't blame me if this chapter puts a dent in the substantial business empires of many. After receiving Aatma Yoga, I incubated upon it for 30 years. Did all the tests, talking and experimentations to first become definite myself. Now I bring Aatma Yoga to you in the most straightforward way possible after trying upon myself and others.

Chapter 4

WHO AM I

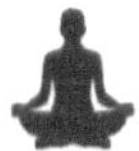

Knowing what you want and who you are is only the beginning of all that Aatma Yoga is. So let us do another small task. Here is a questionnaire about knowing yourself. It's time for you to get clear to yourself about the most important person you have in your life: You.

Tick your area of interest. Also, tick those that talk about your inner feelings that you want to know or find the secrets of ~

- ☐ The goal of my own soul
- ☐ What I am searching in life
- ☐ How to get true love in life
- ☐ How to handle my own sufferings
- ☐ How to end other people's sufferings
- ☐ How to live a life that even my enemies praise me
- ☐ How to die peacefully
- ☐ How to help people to die with peace
- ☐ How to rise above the obstacles that became a routine in my life
- ☐ How to be spiritually at peace
- ☐ How to get over of a particular sin or bad thing I have done in life
- ☐ How to get the good spirits of the world help me succeed
- ☐ How to get true love in life
- ☐ How to never be depressed in life
- ☐ How to be at peace with people that matter to you

- ☐ who am I
- ☐ How to end the circle of life and deaths for my soul
- ☐ How to get the best partner in life
- ☐ How to get the best job/work of your choice in life
- ☐ The difference between human life and all other lives
- ☐ How to make myself happy within
- ☐ How to live a life of content
- ☐ How to get a better next life
- ☐ How to get over my guilt, which I did in the past
- ☐ The ways to give me a never-ending Joy
- ☐ How to handle depression
- ☐ How to bring peace to the lives of friends, family, relatives, etc.
- ☐ human life and its aim
- ☐ The aim of all other life forms
- ☐ How to be at peace when in a difficult situation in life
- ☐ How to get what I want in life

Below you will find a list of significant obstacles. Tick the ones you have a problem with.

- ☐ I want to be 'important' and to be admired by others.
- ☐ I am being or have been counseled for psychological problems.
- ☐ I have a desire for importance.
- ☐ I am greedy
- ☐ I have great fears of speaking up or presenting my opinion.
- ☐ I have a problem with jealousy or envy of others.
- ☐ I have a tendency to cheat others.
- ☐ I have lusted for the opposite sex.

- ☐ I have lusted for same-sex.

- ☐ I have lusted for both sexes.

- ☐ I have lusted for the elderly.

- ☐ I have a problem with anxiety. Sometimes I am confused about why I am so anxious, also about little things.

- ☐ I have contemplated suicide on several occasions

- ☐ I like to hear gossip.

- ☐ I can go to any extent to get what I want, even if it hurts someone else.

- ☐ I have a tendency to be self-destructive.

- ☐ Sometimes I find that I cannot control my anger, it seems to explode before I can stop it.

- ☐ I find it hard to believe in the existence of God.

- ☐ I don't like to work very much. I prefer to relax most of the times.

- ☐ I like to be in control. Power is essential to me.

- ☐ I find myself sleeping more than, and I have no desire or motivation to do anything productive.

- ☐ In the past, I was involved in some occult practices (e.g., Séances, witchcraft, black magic, etc.)

- ☐ Often I am overeating.

- ☐ I have been wrongly treated in the past, and I find it hard to be set free of the inner anger remembering it.

- ☐ I have a terrible habit in my life controls me. I try hard, but I feel like a captive in this situation.

- ☐ I am peaceful in my life and content to remain as I am. I am pretty much happy.

- ☐ I have done drugs

- ☐ I do drugs

☐ I have a hard time with a sex problem. I could never break its control and the bad habits that go with it.

☐ I often feel that my desire for money and possessions has robust control over me.

☐ I find myself lying so that I can impress other people.

☐ Illicit sex

☐ I love Meat-eating

☐ I feel I cannot give up meat eating.

☐ I am whimsical, I like to do what I want when I want to. I don't like to follow the rules and regulations.

☐ Gambling

☐ I have been abused physically, mentally, or emotionally.

☐ I constantly dislike myself.

Chapter 5

WHAT IS AATMA YOGA

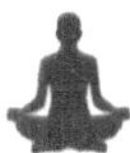

Hey, what is your name? Tell me a little about you. What would be your answer?

I cannot hear your answers, unless you are sitting next to me and tell me about you, in a language I understand well. Let's assume you know all the answers and now, repeat the answers once again, please.

What's your name? Please tell me a little more about yourself, generally.

When you tell me your name, it will be the name that people who know you call you with. It would be the name in your school/college/job registers. The name you know as yours is actually your body's identification code. This is for those people who know you externally!

Imagine that somehow you met a man meditating in a remote Himalayan mountain. He neither knows your name nor your country! Being enlightened, he would be able to see you and interact with you not as an external being, but as what you are within. Your inner self.

What Is the Inner Self

You tell me that.

Imagine, there is a handicapped girl with not so good-looking bone structure or face-value. Are you sure she is as ugly (oops sorry) in nature too as she looks? Maybe she is actually a beautiful, kind and genuine person. Or else all good looking and the so-called cool people would be the most fabulous people to be with too!

Has it ever happened to you that all the people around you and all those who know you, they know you fully? Many times even our parents and spouse, who are supposed to know us well, do not know or understand us.

Often we get surprised to know about another side of us, a hidden talent. Sometimes a place we see or a person we meet for the first time, and we feel we know them or have been here before. Sometimes we crave for this one place and long to be there. And then when we arrive there, we get a vibe that we are home.

So we are not one, we are two existence representing one body.

We often realize that we are one person known externally to the world around. And when we feel that no one understands us, means we have another inner personality. This personality is known only to us. Now let us go more in-depth.

This body which we know and deal with externally, is guided by what is briefly called our 'mind.'

The inner body, inner feelings, that we often say coming from our heart is actually the 'soul.' The heart can be easily represented as the 'face' of our soul while the eyes, it's 'windows.'

The 'soul' we all have within us, is the 'all complete,' the 'perfect being,' the 'role model,' the 'all you would ever need.'

Let's come to this term called "Yoga."

Yoga comes from the word 'Yog,' and this is a Sanskrit word. Sanskrit is the mother of all languages on earth. Yoga thus means 'to unite,' 'to yoke' or 'to join,' 'the union.' Yoga is being at equilibrium: a state in which opposing forces or influences are balanced.

This would lead to the meaning of Aatma Yoga.

Aatma is the 'soul' and yoga is 'union/equilibrium.' So Aatma Yoga means your external being or mind's union with your inner being, 'soul.' When in your 'body' and 'mind' is at equilibrium with your 'soul,' that state is Aatma Yoga.

That would be the Trinity within.

I attach a part of an email message I received from a very realized human being from Germany to me. This is about that state of equilibrium or 'yoga' of the Aatma, in his own way. Such a beautiful story of 'feelings.' Since I did not take his permission to attach his mail, so I do not include his body's identification code. He wrote to my soul from his soul:

"Since my days of youth when I first felt my connection to India or maybe: when I first could name my connection to India which for sure goes back for ages, since these days (back in the 1980s) you've been a constant point of my longing, of my knowing about connectedness.

You may know about the old Greek concept of Platoon of the "Souls" as being round and so self-satisfied that the Gods decided to cut them in halves and that since then the "Souls" are longing and searching for their other half.

In my youth, I heavily believed in this concept.

Somewhen around 1993 just before it became fashionable to include gay characters in movies and books I started writing a novel about a young man discovering that his second half was a man, too.

A few years later, I stopped believing in this concept. I rather assume that there are beings we feel closely connected to, with whom we share more than with others – and with whom for that reason, we in one way or another fall in love.

Another aspect: I have the ability to decide on things from the heart or the belly-brain without the ability (or need!) to explain them completely to anybody (including me). Thus it was in 1991 when I took my bicycle and rode to Southern France (I had never done a similar thing before).

When reaching Arles (where Vincent van Gogh spent some years), I felt that this was the "aim" of this journey. I didn't know this before but it felt like home in a way that I wrote in my diary: "I might never come back here, but I would love to die here" – meaning in some distant future, but on the following evening I was shot by somebody with a gun, just for fun as I assume. I could have been dead but wasn't, and this was up to make more sense of my life from now on.

In 1999 I decided to go to India. I couldn't explain why, I only knew that I wanted to reach out to this vast country with all its colors in culture, languages, music, nature, people, religions, architecture. So 2000 saw me as a traveler, never staying long anywhere (except for Navi Mumbai and Kolkata) on a quest to the "inside" of this my other home country.

I remember the first steps on Indira Gandhi International Airport in February, exhaling the sigh: "ah, finally!" with the sudden feeling of being at home.

And then at Nirmal Hriday around four months later seeing you, hearing your voice throughout this one workday there and all the time trying to grasp the thought: "I know this voice! Where do I know this voice from?" Not so much later it occurred to me natural that you were the reason for my long travel.

I'm sure I told you this story before – as I have told this to quite a few people through the last two decades. For me, it's only logical that we spent more than a workday together before this reunion in a former lifetime.

We have a special connection, so special that it occurs so natural to me that it stayed on and on through the years – a fact that amazes quite some people."

Here are some other words and feelings:

Paramatma:

This is the most beautiful term for any human being. You know the meaning of Aatma, as mentioned before. Now Paramatma is a combination of two words 'Param,' which means highest or supreme and 'Aatma,' you are aware. So Paramatma is the highest inner being/soul.

Saints make it unattainable or very difficult for general people to know or understand Paramatma. This is due to possessiveness/greed/thinking the listener would not appreciate. Paramatma is actually the most simple term/feeling to understand.

So as I mentioned earlier that the first step is to put your finger on the inner you. All answers, all solutions, all that you seek and all your destinations are within 'you.' After that realization, you go about knowing that "all."

How can you have the 'all' and still feel assaulted by the problems and the sufferings? It is simple, you have it all, but you do not know it, and it's 'worth'!

Imagine, you knew you were a musician within but never cared for. And you never did anything about it for a lot part of your life. Suddenly one day by some situation you were forced in a case. And you created music, and your filmmaker friend used it in his film. Then one day you came to know that your music won an Oscar! Suddenly, everyone is taking your inner musician being severe.

We have Paramatma within us always, but mostly, we don't care or don't want to accept it. Or even told that a God or an Allah lives apart from us. Accept that the Almighty resides within you and your life will: Change!

Vhavsagar Paar:

This is another wonder-word from the oldest perfect-language of earth, Sanskrit. This has three words, namely, Vhav, Sagar, and Paar.

See how beautiful this is: 'Vhav' means feelings/emotions, and 'Sagar' means the sea. So Vhavsagar means the sea of emotions/feelings. This we go through in our entire lives, get assaulted by and enjoy in our whole life.

All our emotions get expressed in our thoughts. And the ideas are born in our mind, the ruler of our physical self. So how pleasant and straightforward is Vhavsagar Paar! You know why? Because 'paar' means to 'cross over.'

How do you cross over the constraint of mind towards your Aatma or soul and eventually to the Paramaatma'? You will do that making your 'body' a 'ship/boat' with the sail of your 'mind' to push and steer you, to your destination.

So Aatma Yoga is:

   i. To use your body →

   ii. To cross the obstacle of your mind →

iii. To be in equilibrium with your soul →

iv. To the target the Paramatma, the Supreme Soul.

How simple! Just a few steps more to go from stage i. to reach stage iv. And they would be detailed in the further chapters.

Guna:

Now the most exciting part of this book. Whatever we do or whatever problems we face, depends on the type of people we are. Also what we keep ourselves as and those we meet or interact with.

People have some inherent qualities. So 'guna' would mean 'quality' which some people would be successful in hiding or getting over with. But if you know the various traits, then you would just catch him or know who you are.

In the next chapter, there is a guide for you to check out what your human quality is. We could do something constructive upon us, only when we know ourselves well. There are three essential qualities of a human being that we all would deal with in our day to day life, and also in the mirror.

Tamasik (Evilish): They who just follow the dictates of their body, animal-like.

Rajasik (Middle Path/Hypocrisy): They who follow the dictates of their mind, lower-human like.

Satwik (Role Models): They who lead their lives towards Paramatma like ideal-humans/humane.

Chapter 6

KNOW YOUR SQ

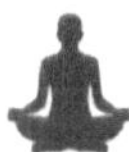

Our Soul is the most important thing we have, so let's nurture it with utmost care.

It's old fashioned to know your IQ, the intelligence quotient. Here your mind and memory is the measure/worth of "yours." That's not the accountability of a human being! That would be a test towards being machines or supercomputers!

Machines, supercomputers, intelligent robots, humanoids, AI, all are great and can serve humans well. But they are just man-made machines created to do specific memory-driven works! Man can make many great things, but not a Soul-Aatma or a Paramatma. Man's mind still cannot conquer over the mysteries of Paramatma and the Aatma. Cannot capture the secrets of life and death and many many similar things. So how can he design one?

High IQ men can artificially help start the creation process. But not the real creating a body, with an intelligent but highly limited mind. Forget creating the Soul. But man can never realize that with even the highest IQ!

But a man who is in the higher stages of Aatma Yoga can do more wonders than anyone can imagine. We can do anything when we can decode the secrets within our own, by ourselves, with Aatma Yoga.

For this, we need to know our SQ, the **Soul Quotient**.

Following is a chart to find out our Inner constitution. Choose a, b or c for the one that describes you well. Be truthful to yourself because who knows your inner self more than you do. Tick in the boxes attached.

1. Cleanliness

- ☐ a. High
- ☐ b. Moderate
- ☐ c. Low

2. Anger

- ☐ a. Rarely
- ☐ b. Sometimes
- ☐ c. Frequently

3. Preferred Drinks

- ☐ a. Water, freshly prepared spices/fruits/vegetable juices
- ☐ b. Tea/coffee/addictives
- ☐ c. Alcohol and its other forms

4. Smoking

- ☐ a. None
- ☐ b. Limited
- ☐ c. Addicted

5. Most Important for You

- ☐ a. Soul
- ☐ b. Mind
- ☐ c. Body

6. Your Choice of Music

- ☐ a. Peaceful
- ☐ b. Loud
- ☐ c. Provocative

7. Personal Nature

- ☐ a. Peaceful
- ☐ b. Gets upset easily
- ☐ c. Agitated

8. Marriage

- ☐ a. Bachelor/one or sex-less marriage/s at a time
- ☐ b. Just the one wife and or prostitutes
- ☐ c. Divorces/many marriages/extra-marital affairs

9. Truthfulness

- ☐ a. Always
- ☐ b. Mostly
- ☐ c. Rarely

10. Work

- ☐ a. Selfless
- ☐ b. For personal goals
- ☐ c. Lazy

11. Pride

- ☐ a. Modest
- ☐ b. Ego
- ☐ c. Vain

12. Children

- ☐ a. All children are my responsibility
- ☐ b. Only my sperm/ova children are mine
- ☐ c. No children my responsibility, not even my own

13. Opposite-sex for Sex

☐ a. Stay away

☐ b. Husband-wife relation and/or prostitutes

☐ c. Objects of necessity, get every woman if possible

14. Enthusiasm

☐ a. Always

☐ b. Sometimes

☐ c. None

15. Doctor Visit

☐ a. Rarely

☐ b. Once a month

☐ c. Often

16. Mind

☐ a. Steady

☐ b. Wants new sensations & variety

☐ c. Wasting time in useless things

17. Creativity

☐ a. Highly

☐ b. Sometimes

☐ c. None

18. Dealing with Personal Problems

☐ a. They know it will become fine

☐ b. Inpatient & inconsistence

☐ c. Blame others

19. Libido

☐ a. Very high but under control

☐ b. Moderate

☐ c. Uncontrollably high

20. Sexual Preference

☐ a. None/homosexual/hetrosexual

☐ b. Hetrosexual+

☐ c. Bisexual +

21. Depression

☐ a. Never

☐ b. Sometimes

☐ c. Frequently

22. Food

☐ a. Eating to survive

☐ b. Loves to eat

☐ c. Survive to eat

23. Food Choice

☐ a. Whole grains/legumes/fresh-fruits/vegetables

☐ b. Fried/spicy/cold drinks/junk/stimulants/addictive

☐ c. Spoiled/chemically treated/processed/refined food

24. Language

☐ a. Uniting everyone

☐ b. My language best for me

☐ c. Force it upon others

25. Violent Behaviour

☐ a. Never

☐ b. Sometimes

☐ c. Frequently

26. Seeks

☐ a. Joy

☐ b. Happiness

☐ c. Pleasures

27. Strangers

☐ a. Welcome

☐ b. Avoid

☐ c. Upsetting to confront

28. Quarreling

☐ a. Avoid

☐ b. Sometimes

☐ c. Always ready

29. Fighting

☐ a. Never

☐ b. Avoid

☐ c. Always ready

30. Inner Thoughts

☐ a. Selfless

☐ b. Selfish

☐ c. Destructive

31. Psychological Blockage

- ☐ a. Harmonious & adaptable
- ☐ b. Finds defects of others
- ☐ c. Deep-seated blockage

32. New Things

- ☐ a. Happy to know
- ☐ b. Ok, if I have to
- ☐ c. No need

33. Pray/Puja/Namaj

- ☐ a. Never but respects
- ☐ b. Occasionally
- ☐ c. Have to do

34. All other living beings are

- ☐ a. My family, for us to serve them
- ☐ b. Use them as required
- ☐ c. Their lives are unworthy/soulless/for our use/consumption

35. I earn money for

- ☐ a. Selfless Works
- ☐ b. Family, friends and relatives
- ☐ c. Me

36. I Donate

- ☐ a. 90% +
- ☐ b. 0 – 90%
- ☐ c. 0 or to show off

37. Spiritual Study

☐　a. Daily

☐　b. Occasionally

☐　c. Never

38. Convert/Change people's way

☐　a. Fool-proof/giving people personal examples of goodness

☐　b. Stay the way born thoughtlessly

☐　c. Forced/greedy/helpless and fool-through conversions

39. Serve Self-Country

☐　a. Daily

☐　b. Frequently

☐　c. Rarely

40. Need for Sleep

☐　a. Little

☐　b. Moderate

☐　c. High

41. Forgiveness

☐　a. Easily

☐　b. With efforts

☐　c. Holds grudges

42. Peace of Mind

☐　a. Generally

☐　b. Partly

☐　c. Rarely

43. Drug/Alcohol/Stimulant

- ☐ a. Never
- ☐ b. Occasionally
- ☐ c. Frequently

44. Life

- ☐ a. Optimist
- ☐ b. Just exist
- ☐ c. Pessimist

45. Generally

- ☐ a. Fearless
- ☐ b. Restless
- ☐ c. Depressed

46. Kaliyug, the present-day Dark Age

- ☐ a. End in Kaliyug
- ☐ b. Survival in Kaliyug
- ☐ c. Cause of Kaliyug

47. Humanity

- ☐ a. My life is dedicated to Humanity's benefit
- ☐ b. Just Self
- ☐ c. Destruction of Humanity

48. Earn

- ☐ a. To share with others
- ☐ b. To spend on self and family and share a little
- ☐ c. For personal luxury only

49. Good Actions

☐ a. Continuous striving to better, selflessly

☐ b. Lacks it unless required for a benefit

☐ c. Just to get/snatch/lure converts

50. For Nature

☐ a. Adds/creates

☐ b. Let's nature to be as it is

☐ c. Destroyer of nature

51. Attachment to Money

☐ a. Little, for basic requirements only

☐ b. Yes, to save for later

☐ c. A lot, madness

52. Energy and Emotions

☐ a. Rejuvenated and always full

☐ b. Limited

☐ c. Stagnant and repressed

53. Problems in Life

☐ a. Solved

☐ b. What to do

☐ c. Complain about them but still stay thus

54. They accept their conditions in Life as

☐ a. Passing

☐ b. Fight it

☐ c. Fate

55. Allow Negative Influences to

- ☐ a. Never come near
- ☐ b. Fight them
- ☐ c. Dominated by them

56. People of other religions/sects

- ☐ a. Love all, as they are your own spiritual siblings
- ☐ b. Their authority says they are lesser/convert them
- ☐ c. Their authority says convert them or kill them

57. To be part of their Religion

- ☐ a. You are born as the Almighty wanted, perfect
- ☐ b. You choose what you get by birth
- ☐ c. Do something external/unnatural to convert them

58. Love

- ☐ a. Universal
- ☐ b. Personal
- ☐ c. None

59. Contentment

- ☐ a. Usually
- ☐ b. Partly
- ☐ c. Never

60. Use of Truth

- ☐ a. Practice by all means
- ☐ b. Truth and lies depending on personal needs
- ☐ c. Just Lies

61. Beauty

☐ a. Inner beauty

☐ b. External show-offs

☐ c. Involuntarily spreading ugliness

62. Love is

☐ a. Selfless loving

☐ b. Selfish loving

☐ c. Just love me

63. Dealing with Personal Problems

☐ a. They know it will become fine

☐ b. Inpatient & Inconsistence

☐ c. Blame others

64. Character

☐ a. Never forget good deeds of others

☐ b. Forgets good acts of others

☐ c. Always looks for a chance to revenge

65. Serve Humanity

☐ a. Daily

☐ b. Occasionally

☐ c. Never

66. Highest for me is

☐ a. Spirituality

☐ b. Family

☐ c. Me

67. Speech

- ☐ a. Calm & peaceful
- ☐ b. Agitated
- ☐ c. Dull & upsetting

68. Concentration

- ☐ a. Good
- ☐ b. Moderate
- ☐ c. Poor

69. Food

- ☐ a. Super-veg/vegetarian/vegan
- ☐ b. Non-veg with restraint
- ☐ c. Non-veg without restraint/eats anything that moves

70. For the weak and unable

- ☐ a. Protects them
- ☐ b. Stays away from them
- ☐ c. Attack/kill/destroys them

71. Motivation

- ☐ a. Balance of social duties and personal rights
- ☐ b. Personal rights mostly
- ☐ c. Just personal gains and society be damned

72. Faith in Goodness and the Almighty

- ☐ a. Total
- ☐ b. Doubtful
- ☐ c. No faith/slavery/sheep-like following

73. Life is

- ☐ a. Passionately living
- ☐ b. Just existing in life
- ☐ c. Life is hell/make life hell for others

74. Mind

- ☐ a. Steady
- ☐ b. Wants new sensations & variety
- ☐ c. Wasting time in useless things

75. Women for you

- ☐ a. The creators, most respectable
- ☐ b. They must try to be equal, but must never succeed
- ☐ c. Lower beings, only good for baby production, use and throw

76. Will Power

- ☐ a. Strong
- ☐ b. Variable
- ☐ c. Weak

77. Sensory Impressions

- ☐ a. Calm & Pure
- ☐ b. Mixed
- ☐ c. Disturbed

78. Fear

- ☐ a. Rarely
- ☐ b. Sometimes
- ☐ c. Frequently

79. Character

☐ a. Never forget good deeds of others

☐ b. Forgets good acts of others

☐ c. Always looks for a chance to revenge

80. Personal Hygiene

☐ a. Always fresh

☐ b. Hide

☐ c. Poor

81. Problems in Life

☐ a. Solved

☐ b. What to do

☐ c. Do not know

82. They accept their Conditions in Life as

☐ a. Passing

☐ b. Fight

☐ c. Fate

83. Allow Negative Influences to

☐ a. Never come near

☐ b. Fight them

☐ c. Dominate them

84. Baby Producing

☐ a. Without touching opposite sex

☐ b. Controlled production using rubbers

☐ c. Uncontrolled/produces bastards/murders self-babies

85. Memory

- ☐ a. Good
- ☐ b. Moderate
- ☐ c. Poor

86. Control of Senses

- ☐ a. Good
- ☐ b. Moderate
- ☐ c. Weak

87. The desire for external things

- ☐ a. Little
- ☐ b. Frequent
- ☐ c. Excessive

88. Relation with God

- ☐ a. Within them and body is temple
- ☐ b. Religious by need/greed
- ☐ c. Killing in the name of religion

89. Religion

- ☐ a. Dharma (living for others, binds/balances the universe)
- ☐ b. External God kept outside of self
- ☐ c. Fear generating anti-divine but showing off as God-lover

90. Gambling/Lottery

- ☐ a. Never
- ☐ b. Sometimes/occationally
- ☐ c. Often/mostly

Now you have to send me the answer sheet. Just kidding! You do not need me or anyone to know your self. You would be able to do much better with yourself.

All you have to do is,

i. Count all the 'a' in your answers and multiply that number with 2

ii. Count all the 'b' in your answers and multiply that number with 1

iii. Count all the 'c' in your answers and multiply that number with −2

For example in your total answers, you had 25 'a,' 35 'b' and 25 'c,' so the result will be from $25 \times 2 = 50$, $35 \times 1 = 35$ and $25 \times -2 = -50$.

Thus your SQ will be: $50 + 35 - 50 = 35$ simple mathematics.

Highest score available is 180

Least score you can get is −180

And you will know what is your Soul's Quotient SQ according to this:

Score: 160 through 180: You are a Kohinoor

Score: 120 through 160: You are a Satwik

Score: 000 through 120: You are a Rajasik

Score: −100 through 000: You are a Tamasik

Score: −180 through −100: You are a Devil

If you are a Kohinoor, then please come and meet me as soon as possible. If you are a Satwik, then how beautiful it is for the entire humanity to have you. And how beautiful it will be to meet you here at your Satwik Humane Abode, Hari Dhaam in Kolkata, INDIA.

For others, please strive to be a Satwik, it would be effortless. I would be happy to guide you towards becoming a Satwik. Be our SoulDost and contact me, and we will take the next step from there on.

Chapter 7

EXPLANATIONS
AND POST DEATH

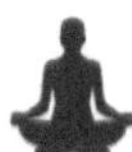

In 2002 I started my Satwik Gurukuls. They are the immaculate knowledge centers which do not run on taking fees from the students. Nor by taking grants/donations/charity/handouts from governments. Also not by NGOs/foreign agencies/mafias/religious organizations etc.

How then does it run? Because the teachers/staff/essentials/food/hostel etc. everything needs to be paid! Such a Satwik Gurukul runs by three forces:

One is selfless love oriented management given by Korak Day.

Secondly, sharing like you are doing that for your own family. This is every month, with responsibility. Also, with the feeling that all the people you are serving are your own soul-family. This is a responsibility you must take for your entire life like Dr. Dipak N Patel from the USA did. Even Korak Day's parents did that too, with their own limitations.

Thirdly the prayers/blessings given by those who wanted such an epoch to succeed.

I could have accepted donations from the Governments too, but I didn't! The governments actually looted from me instead. Doing for the unprivileged and the destitute is the government's responsibility. Since our start in 2002, we did not have spiritually healthy governments in Bengal where we started, nor in India. So there was no one in politics to appreciate the potential of this work. Nor do we have in Bengal a caring government, even now in 2019. The central government is truthful, but king Modi is still very busy.

All the countries have equal responsibility for the unprivileged humans anywhere on earth.

A Satwik Aacharay is a selfless teacher. He transfers all the knowledge his soul has to his students, not for money but as a humane responsibility. Shishyays are the students who do not buy a teacher. But they give their truthful soul to be knowledgable. A Satwik Gurukul is thus an abode of such knowledge transfers.

In my Satwik Gurukul, one day as the Shishyays were attentive to their Satwik Aacharay, this beautiful thing happened:

"Aacharay why some people are born as destitute, some are born to the Billionaires? Some people are ascetics, some as terrorists," said Jamal, a Shishyay.

"Why some are born as a cow and murdered while some are born as a whale in the Pacific Ocean reaching a cooking pot? Some as crows disliking all other birds and some as a maggot eating rotten flesh," asked Rashid.

"Why some people become ghosts after death and some glow with light on death," asked Javed.

"What is Paap (the result of doing bad things) and what is Punya (the result of doing good things)," asked Nitai.

A younger Shishyay Shabbir, who was staring at the elder Shaishyays, suddenly spoke out, "let's go play."

"Shut up and sit quietly," shouted Muzammil.

"But I don't understand what you all are saying!"

Aacharay, "Sit down, Muzammil, I will tell you an interesting story first."

Jamal, "But what about our questions, Aacharay?"

"Your answers will be there in the story."

There was a beautiful Pine tree covered hills of the Himalayas in Darjeeling, India. A tiny village was there which had two families who lived nearby. For many kilometers there lived no one else. They were poor and survived on very less money. One family had a mother and her 6 years old son whose father left them to get remarried to a rich girl in Nepal.

Another family had an elderly couple whose only son worked in a far off Indian city Bangalore. He was a security guard and lived there with his family. He would send some money every month to his father, on which the elderly couple would survive.

The young mother Prabha would work at the nearby tea garden. There she would get a minimal amount of 110 Rupees, and thus she took care of her son, Jivan.

The man Dadu of the elderly couple loved little Jivan very much. Prabha would leave Jivan with Dadu whenever she went for plucking tea leaves in the Tea Garden. The boy was very naughty and of course, didn't like to go to a school, in another village.

Little Jiwan and Dadu would often play a game.

Dadu had many Thulo Olaichi (big-cardamom) shrubs and Ruk-Tamatar (tree tomatoes) trees around his hut.

"Whenever you will do something good, I will give you a Thulo Olaichi, and if you do something 'very' good, I will give to 4. You will keep them on the shade of your hut. And if you do something wrong, I will provide you with a Ruk-Tamatar while if you do something 'very' wrong, then I will give you 4. You will keep them in different ditches in the ground, nearby your hut and mark them. When there is an emergency, and you urgently need money, you can get a lot of money selling the Ruk-Tamattars and the Thulo Olaichis."

This way, the time went on. Both Dadu and Jivan enjoyed their game.

Whenever Jivan would do something right, he would get 1 or 4 Thulo Olaichi. As he would do bad things like not listening to his mother. Also, when he did not reply when called, would not eat lunch, etc., he would get 1 or 4 Ruk-Tamatars.

Often Jivan thought that Dadu is foolish to give him 4 Ruk-Tamatars when he would do nasty things.

Four years passed, and Jivan was 10 years old now. A tourist felt unconscious nearby his house. This happened when he was tracking on the nearby mountains. Jivan shouted and called Dadu for help. He brought water and washed his wound and his head.

He took very excellent care of the tourist. Soon within three days the tourist from Israel got well, thanked them, and went his way. That day Dadu called Jivan and gave him 30 Ilaichis.

"Why so many, Dadu?"

"Because you did a very very good thing by saving the life of a human being."

That same night when Prabha returned from the Tea Garden, she was very sick, with a high fever. She came home and slept with many blankets over her. Dadu asked Jiwan to make a Khichari of boiled rice and daal.

Jivan made the Khichari and fed his mother, but she ate a little and slept again. The whole night Jivan changed water-soaked cloth. He kept it on her forehead, to reduce her temperature.

Nothing changed, and in the morning, Prabha was sicker.

Dadu advised Jivan to go to nearby Sukhia Pokhari Market and get the government doctor.

"You would need a lot of money there to bring the doctor here. So take your Ruk-Tamatars and Thulo Olaichi and sell them off at the Friday market today. Use the money for the doctor and the medicines. You sure have a lot of them both by now."

He first went to dig up the Tomatoes because he knew he had more tomatoes than the cardamoms. He dug the ground and in one place and then another location and then other. But there was nothing, except for some bad stuff!

He shouted, "Dadu see what has happened to all my Ruk-Tamatars. They are all rotten!" Dadu came hurried, "oh, all are rotten?"

"yes, Dadu!"

"Yes, they were the fruits of bad actions you did, so they will always be rotten and of no use to you. Bad actions will give you big results, I mean big fruits, but soon they will rot and become useless!"

"Dadu I must check the Thulo Olaichi, maybe they too are rotten!"
Jivan runs, keeping Dadu smiling. He goes slowly towards the direction
Jivan went.

Jivan was astonished to see all the cardamoms to be ripe and dry,
best quality. He looks at Dadu, and Dadu smiles back. Jiwan puts them
in a cloth and tie that and put on a stick end.

"Now go fast and sell them in the Haat market. Then use the money
for the doctor, run" Jivan runs in the thin curving village mud road. He
carries his cardamoms in a cloth bundle on a stick end.

In the Haat, he was trying to sell the Cardamoms, but he was not
getting a reasonable price. Just then the Israeli tourist who was also
there taking pictures, saw Jivan.

"Hey Jivan, what are you doing here?"

Jivan put his little palm on his forehead, "Mother is sick, and I am
trying to sell them to get money for the doctor and the medicines." His
Nepali guide translates that to the tourist, Nityanhu. His eyes get filled
with tears so much that they flow down his cheeks.

He asks the translator to translate, "I will buy them, how much?"

"$10 only."

"But they are so fresh and smell so good I will give $500 for them as
I just have that much cash now with me."

Jivan nods his head, "no, only $10."

"But why? You saved my life, and I want to thank you."

"No my Dadu says not to accept anything in return for the good
things you do for others. Because then you will get rotten Ruk-Tamatars
which actually turn useless."

Nityanhu gives him $10 and takes all the cardamoms from him.
Jivan runs to the doctor. Nityanhu too runs behind him.

The doctor is reluctant to go.

"Take this money and please come and save my mother, I have no
one else on earth. You have to save my mother, please, doctor!"

"Doctor, you have to go and save his mother, whatever money it takes, I will give you! Hurry up, get an ambulance, now!! And mind it, this child must know that it's his money which is doing all this." He says and then stops his Nepali guide as he was going to translate it. "Robin stop, he knows English."

Jivan is a common name in Indian, and Jivan means 'life.'

Aacharay, "Did you like the story, Muzammil?"

"Aacharay, my father has also left my mother and 4 sisters of mine and married some Chinal whore in Mallikpur." Aacharay hushes him and tells him not to use such words. Muzammil looks blankly at his Aacharay, whom he loves a lot.

"Aacharay, what about our questions then?" asked Javed.

"Simple answer, my dear! When we do good things we get 'plus' points, the more the good, the more 'plus' points we get. You know everything is pre-decided as how many 'plus' points you will get for which good thing you did.

Similarly, when you do bad things, you get 'minus' points. Worse stuff you do, the higher 'minus' points for you! This will continue throughout your life's journey!

When you die, all your plus points are added and also your minus points.

Say you accumulated +1 million points in your whole life doing various good works/actions. At the same time, you collected −5 million points, similarly by doing a lot of bad things.

So your total will be −4 Million. Awful show! So what do you expect to get?"

Many fool-through present day enslaving groups and establishments called religions or political party would tell you:

☐ Follow my group's authority, and all your sins will vanish.

☐ Do/give this and your sins and evil actions would vanish.

☐ Go and bathe in this river and drink this well's water etc. and all, vanish.

- ☐ Pay this much amount and, vanish.

- ☐ Do this kind of fasting for this duration and, vanish.

- ☐ Eat in this person's home and all your good, vanish.

- ☐ Hate this person's birth-life and your sins, vanish.

- ☐ Murder this and that animal in my group's way and, vanish.

- ☐ Blast these innocent humans, and all your greeds would be fulfilled.

- ☐ Get yourself killed, and in heaven, your desires would be fulfilled.

- ☐ Do this kind of breathing exercise and, vanish.

- ☐ Go to this building and, vanish.

- ☐ Fight wars in my group's greed and fulfill your greeds and, vanish.

I could add here so many more such slave-orders for the slaves of such groups. I also know that you could add much more than I could. You got the point, isn't it? Newton's Third Law mentions that every action has an equal and opposite reaction. This is true in all fields related to humans, and for everything on earth.

Now we come to the **Soul Actions Post Death.**

In the final moments of your death and after your breathing stops, the following happens:

Step #1 Pran Ganit (Life Math Calculations):

All your "+" and the "−" points are calculated of our life works/ thoughts/actions et all. Then the results are declared. According to the results, the soul is designated to its destination.

Step #2 Aatma Gati (Soul's Destinations):

A. Urdhava Gati: Movement to other worlds.

1. Satwik Tangencials: Parmatma Prapti (become one with the Almighty), Devine Abode.

2. Rajasik Tangencials: Pitrilok Prapti (attachment to the body lasts), Ghost Life.

3. Tamasik Tangencials: Hell.

B. Sthir Gati: Movement again to the same Human Womb.

1. Satwik Human Births: Born as an enlightened soul and lives a Saintly life.

2. Rajasik Human Births: Born in a family of happiness and enjoyable life.

3. Tamasik Human Births: Born in a poor/destitute womb with sad/scarcity-filled life.

C. Adho Gati: Movement to the Lower-Life Wombs.

1. Satwik Lower Births: Trees, Cows, animals, birds, fishes, etc. who serve humanity closely.

2. Rajasik Lower Births: Trees, animals, birds, fishes, etc. who serve humanity partially.

3. Tamasik Lower Births: Insects, reptiles, non-moving lives, animals, birds, etc. who harms humanity.

Step #3: Assignments:

1. Satwik Tangencials: Pran Ganit is more than "+ Koti" (10 Million). GOD

2. Satwik Human Births: Pran Ganit is more than "+ Laksh" (100,000).

3. Rajasik Human Births: Pran Ganit is more than "+ Ayut" (10,000).

4. Tamasik Human Births: Pran Ganit is more than "+ Sata" (100).

5. Rajasik Tangencials: Pran Ganit is "Zero." GHOST

6. Satwik Lower Births: Pran Ganit is less than "− Sata" (100).

7. Rajasik Lower Births: Pran Ganit is less than "− Ayut" (10,000).

8. Tamasik Lower Births: Pran Ganit is less than "− Laksh" (100,000).

9. Tamasik Tangencials: Pran Ganit is less than "− Koti" (10 Million). HELL

This is just an introduction to the whole after-death soul-movements. Also, please note that the assignments in step three vary in case of the different cycles of time. The above assignments are according to Pran Ganit is in the times of Kaliyug. Kaliyug is the present times of destruction, darkness, and evil). It differs in Dwapar Yug, Treta Yug and the best in the Golden Age (Satyug).

This Golden Age, Satyug, is the mission of all Satwiks and those who practice Aatma Yoga.

Before closing this chapter, one thing is clear that all the bad and the good we get is what we have earned. The more we want to change our bad life to a good life, the more we got to gather the + points in life by doing positive actions, Su-karm.

Chapter 8

WHAT PEOPLE FELT

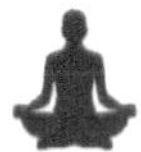

Some Souls shares their Struggles/Thanks/Hopes with the Satwik Aacharay Korak Day. This relates to the topic of this book. Souls have no names and as they are souls who shared with a soul who is in resonance with Aatma-Yoga. So their names are kept away, and only the names of their countries/cities are mentioned here:

- ❑ "We all made you our 'Ideal' – which we would strive to raise our standards, to behave in the way you followed every minute of every day. That's how we saw you. Korak made the concept of 'sweet sacrifice' so real, we said... Meeting you has been the most important, religious and educational experience of my life." DM, Retired Principal, **Dublin**

- ❑ "They say going to India can change a person's life," I feel this is true to a large extent. Similarly, for me, you are a large part of that – you are an important part of India. Many people say, 'Korak you are not Indian' but you embody the essence of India, too. Strong Faith and Deep beliefs. You are deep and complex...just like India's massive culture." MP, **Hollywood**

- ❑ "I have come to see the 'epicenter of life' my own thoughts are that the epicenter of life is where the Spirit of Living exists in its overwhelming fullness...the spirit exists so fully in You." A, Lawyer, **Singapore**

- ❑ "There's something about children eyes: they are so lightning, illuminated with wonders, Joy...and when they turn 15 years old, this light usually becomes harder to see...but you managed to keep the light, don't lose it!!!" CD, **France**

- "Thank you for teaching me the importance of being human first, then being a doctor" **English** Doctor

- "I always asked God to make his presence felt and through you, I felt him." Film Actress and Dancer, **Kolkata**

- "Dear Korak I am deeply touched by your mode of thinking. I wholly agree with you that the number of years a person lives in this world is of no consequence whether to him or to the world. But even a day spent in true service of mankind is supreme and of any importance... I have this thinking that definitely an old person can talk about ideologies and Godly ways with ease. But since you are young and yet so modest, I am able to accept your thoughts more comfortably." JM, **Assam Girl**

- "Br. Korak, the wise sage...has been like a guru to me; a sweet, dear friend, a tough compassionate 'boss.'" ML, Faith Mag, **USA**

- "My Mother gave birth to me. You gave me life. I was in a womb for the last 24 years and everything that has ever happened to me was essential, as everything that happens in the womb of a mother is essential for growth. But it was your love that took me out of the womb and now I can crawl. Without love, there is no life." DP, Doctor, **USA**

- "Truthfully, you're amazing Korak. Oh I know it is all God's will but it takes much effort, dedication and suffering from you for that to happen. I wish I could be more like you. I'm going to try though. I'm being tested now more than ever before in my life... Doing all my work is very hard under these circumstances, but I find if I think of you, then this helps inspire me to keep going. So thank you, my dear friend, for being you." PS, **England**

- "You know me well. Give me your precious advice. Thank you Korak, You are my Soul friend." F, **Belgium**

- "I enjoy the wisdom that you write about and it helps to hear someone speak with wisdom about truth and love and speak of God." D, **USA**

- "Thank you for the time that you've spent, making me improve myself." J, **Montreal**

- "My friend I love you and I know how beautiful your soul is. Any hurt I felt was in part because of my difficult relationship with my soul, which wants so much that it does not have and isn't satisfied by the things I do have, so I become frustrated that I have not brought my life and my soul's desire together. So this story repeats over and over, sometimes I do not want this soul, I want one that is easier to please, perhaps I am saying I sometimes wish not to be me. I feel trapped by everything I should do, by the idea of success itself. I want to drop out of this striving for success for its own sake, I want to try less to do those things that I should do and try more to do those things that I most want. But my life seems to be dominated by these lifeless forms that I care little about so that there is no time to really feel I am alive." JB, **Wisconsin**

- "You are the only friend I have who offers me constructive criticism, offers me your feelings on what areas I can improve myself, and who doesn't flatter me. Who wants the best for me." DP, **New York**

- "In Spain, the people and me also are dirthi inside is very difficult to find the magic and the beauty of the things. Yes, yes, im know the beauty is inside myself but im only small animal but I try to...ok sorry for my small and stupits problems please don't lose your beauty and remember im love you, great man." M, **Spain**

- "I know that people are born with deformities and illnesses that last their whole lives. So perhaps this is an illness I have been born with. Or perhaps, as you say, it comes because I have a very special destiny. Even though I am not sure what the truth is, I have faith in you. I have more faith in your advice than in anyone else's. So I will do what you recommend." JB, **USA**

- "Me I am like a wall: unbreakable. Korak always comes back with his pneumatic drill to break the wall, and give light behind this wall." NS, **Paris**

❏ "Thanks for the blessings, Korak. You are in the right place at the right time and God/Allah is using your gifts. Gifts are given away but keep multiplying and returning to you – grander than you ever expect. Love is like that when it is based on God. Keep up the special work." Dr. KB, **US**

❏ "I'm often not good when I speak about you. But last time I was speaking with a friend, I was speaking about your power and determination and I said: "I'm sure Korak understand something we don't know or we don't see or we don't feel." And after half a day I understand that this is the answer to the question: "Why Korak is attracting people?" You know that I have no religion, no spirituality, and no God. So I think there is a message from your soul and your heart that is transformed by your brain in determination and power. I can see that in your body, in your actions, in your words. Your brain is working well like our brain, but your brain is working in the way of your soul and heart (internal), our brain is working in the way of body and visual things (external)." NS, **France**

❏ "It's with a mixture of awe and admiration that I read about the various projects you seem to manage all at the same time. And most of all, I have profound respect for your ability to recognize what's most important: your focus seems always to be on enriching their souls rather than just their bodies." D, **Canada**

❏ "It is so beautiful what you write. It speaks to the soul"! F, **Belgium**

❏ "Your sharing has always touched me deeply. You are remarkable in your willingness to pass on every little bit that God blessed you with. Your friend from **Singapore**, A

❏ "Hi Korak, Today I taught again. The educational system takes the love and beauty out of knowledge and makes it into some requirement and career path...which is often a path to suffering even if it leads to money." J, **USA**

❏ "We are constantly, daily, hourly being reminded and told how great the country is and how fortunate we are and how much we have to be thankful for. In medical school, it seems even more. 'We are fortunate to have this medicine and clean water and this and that and this and that.' Every day this is the message. Even during the bad times, we are programmed to think that it could be worse.' At least we are not in poor countries.' Constantly it is announced how Americans take this and that for granted and how we don't appreciate anything. All the supposedly great things we have of freedom, democracy, opportunities, and choices...all the external prayers are for being thankful for the conveniences and comforts and the life's free from the so-called material hardships. You know about all this...the pity parties and how the rest of the world is supposedly miserable and struggling in their poverty. In such an atmosphere, I think it may backfire to be so direct about internal poverty and where it is and how internal poverty is the true poverty and the poorest of the poor. If we had to admit that the internal poverty is the true poverty and the poorest of the poor live here, it would completely shatter the deeply established illusions of America's greatness and it's people and how the external choices and things are not so important. I don't think people's egos would allow for such a thing, especially not on a large scale of people. Their life would be flipped upside down. If people had to admit that the freedoms and choices are not important to the real, lasting beautiful things in life and that maybe even these external things prevent the deep experiences of beauty and love." D, **USA**

❏ "Korak, You are a genius, man! You told me to take some pictures of my class, and also a picture of me teaching. I did that today when I had a review session for the test. The class really smiled when I did it. Then I asked one student to take a picture of me. Those made the class laugh too. It was wonderful. I love you Korak. So much good advice comes to me through you." J, **USA**

❏ "Take care of yourself. Through you comes to the opportunity for LOVE to spread around the World like a stone thrown into the water that creates ever-widening ripples. These ripples are of LOVE which is there to change Man's attitude to their brothers/Humanity... Keep on creating those ripples"!!!!!
R, **England**

- ❑ "No one else would give me this advice, because everyone is afraid I will suffer the same things again. But if it must come, let it come. I WILL face it. And you are right. I can face it better now than I have in the past. I do not think your advice is funny. Some people close to me would say it is dangerous advice, and that I should seek a professional person, a therapist or psychiatrist to talk to about these issues. Even though I am not sure what the truth is, I have faith in you. I have more faith in your advice than in anyone else's. So I will do what you recommend." J, **USA**

- ❑ "Right now I am living a difficult time, I feel my life is absolutely empty, I'm feeling terribly lonely and useless in this society. I really feel I don't fit in my way of life, my town, my job, my house, and my family and relations don't fulfill my soul. Right now I have a tremendous fight inside myself so I'm feeling I have to return to India and see what to do." Du, **Spain**

- ❑ "I agree with your words whole-heartedly. Some of my best friends are in the WTO and OECD and they just sit around and have extravagant dinner parties and drinks. Action is the key, and you my dear friend, are certainly the man when it comes to that. I've been out of the loop for the past weeks while experiencing the world of yoga up in Rishikesh and doing a ten-day Vipassana meditation retreat which really blew my mind to smithereens. Life IS about love, and that is why your work is so inspiring to me. I want to learn this over the next years of my life as I am only now really just waking up to the suffering all us species go through in our lives." N, **New Zealand**

- ❑ "Last night you talked to Dipak and told him that whatever we do is good and God will have the control of what we say and do, and our efforts are more important than our successes. This helped me so much and made me relax and enjoy doing this good work. I have found the marketing and promotions side of this work to be humbling and difficult for me. It is contrary to my personality to approach people and to try to sell them on these ideas. Also, I find that the motivation for many of the film entries in the festival is less true and pure than your/ our film. This has made me feel vulnerable. I feel that last night at the opening gala was a success. I spoke with many people about the film, about you, and about Aamar Nijer. There were many people who responded positively and I do not know if they were being nice or genuinely interested, but that was not my responsibility. One person expressed that they were interested in our film above all because it was not influenced by the desire for stardom or profit. It was art done through human beings to help the unloved and that really appealed to him. Another person asked me why we did not have a table set up to promote the film. I told her that this was because we did not have the money/felt that it was not a good use of money for what Aamar Nijer is about. She held onto my arm and said that she would love to see a film that is created by people without money and not influenced by such earthly things. I got such a good feeling from being a part of this film above all else at the festival. I learned that details and successes are fine to desire, but love and goodness come from the work itself." S, **LA**

❑ "You have already done enough for me, to last me a lifetime. I don't think anyone will ever be able to do as much for me as you have." DNP, **USA**

❑ "You are promised to do great things for the destitute because you are yourself a destitute of love and you sometimes take the place of a destitute of Kolkata's streets. The world needs you"!!! E, **France**

❑ "The path you have chosen is not the very common only person who has gone through an immense amount of self-realization can think about it. The world is full of people who sleep through their entire life, and believe me the most heinous crime they think is to wake them up nothing can be rewarding in the materialistic sense in this world for this." T, **India**

❑ "I just wanted to let you know that I've thought about you, especially about your wish not to accept charity... I've seen myself that this charity the US and Europe give as development assistance can be a harmful thing... I've seen how some people have no confidence in them and believe they must wait for help from a rich person or country. In Benin, it was hard for me to be a white person there since many people just see that I have money and want me to give them something. I didn't even know if I should be there, for that reason. Maybe I was part of the problem." JB, **USA**

❑ "I am going away for a few days to one of our most Holy shrines, I will have a Mass said especially for you and for your intentions and for your work and will send on the card to you. I spoke to you before about a community of enclosed silent Sisters whom I visit...a good friend of mine many years ago she joined this convent and is still there... they live a silent life of prayer mainly. I have spoken to them about you each time I have come home from Kolkata about Kalighat. The first time I came home two years ago, most of what I said was about you and what so many others and I learned from you and how you inspired so many and how you taught us what it meant to love God by loving our neighbors...the poorest of the poor. So they remembered your name and when I went back to talk to them about my last year's visit, they asked me if Korak was there and how was he, etc. They also saw your film and thought it was beautiful and so meaningful and I gave them your book of poems and writings also which they use regularly among themselves...but the point I want to make is this. One day a young man, about 28 years old called into the convent. Many people call into these convents to talk to the sisters about their lives, or their hopes, or their problems or to ask for prayers to help them with decisions or to ask for advice etc etc... that is their mission...prayer and to be there for anyone who needs them...anyway this Australian called in to talk... I do not know what he wanted to talk about...but imagine the surprise the sister got when he said he had been in Kolkata for a while and had met this extraordinary man called Korak in Kalighat...a man whom he will never forget, a man who inspired him so much...the Sister smiled and told him that she had heard so much about this Korak (from me) from a friend of hers...and so you became a large part of their chat..." DM, **Ireland**

❑ "You know Korak this western society is so different from India. Internal Poverty is everywhere and engulfs people as soon as they are born. For example, we are about to come up to Christmas now. This is the time when all the companies big and small start these relentless advertising campaigns telling people that they must buy everyone something expensive and cool and completely useless to them. If they don't then society has been taught to think that the person is selfish and unworthy and uncaring. Yet every year on Christmas day I go to cook dinner for and spend time with elderly people who have been put in care homes and abandoned by their families. They don't even come to see them on Christmas day and no one forgives each other. Maybe they send these elderly some cool present in the post with a card that says 'Merry Christmas Dad, from Mark.' And Mark thinks "I'm glad that job is out the way now." One thing I keep feeling to share with you is that these societies are a long-time, love-neglected mess. They aren't going to change overnight or with little effort. They start with unhelpful attitudes but you can't tell them that because they don't understand and they might even take offense. You can only shine the beautiful light of your loving and example and they will slowly follow. It's interesting I'm writing this to you, but I'm also writing it to me. I forget sometimes but you keep inspiring and reminding me." P, **London**

❑ "Today, I was studying some physiology, we were studying the kidney section for this last month or so, and I got the feeling that the kidney organ was very much like you. It was small and unnoticed and often overlooked. Most people don't give the kidney much attention nor do they know where the kidney is and couldn't tell you what the kidney does for the body. Yet, the kidney can be the greatest, most important and essential organ of the body. It quietly and humbly does its life-saving work for the body, 365 days a year with not one moment to rest. It is strong, resilient and can withstand the toxic onslaught that it often receives from what people give it. Remove one whole kidney and half the other and still it will carry out its duty. And so it is with you, my friend." D, **USA**

❑ "It's so strange. I never had any culture shock coming to India. I just walked out of Calcutta Airport and smiled to myself and said that I was home. I really felt that. Coming back to Australia, I feel that I don't belong and that I don't want to." TG **Australia**

❑ "We are entering Holy Week: you know how important it is to us: Christ will die on Friday and be raised on Easter Sunday. Through him, mankind (meaning each of us) will be able to see God and share his own life! This deep love in your heart, the one you give to each resident in Kalighat, every volunteer passing by comes from Him. You are giving a true testimony of him living in you, and thus give him to the persons you meet. This is He that I love so much in you, Him hiding in the disguise of a loving Hindu. And through loving deeds, he is giving himself to others through you." Fr.I, **France**

❑ "I am doing fine, but living here in America is still not an easy task. I am not really feeling like I can stay at my dad's house, and I also feel weird living at my mom's house. I must find an apartment before I go insane! If I had a place for myself, anywhere, like a small bedroom where I knew I was welcome, then I would be a lot better off and could start to relax which would be good. Anyways it's all part of the lifestyle in America." SG **USA**

❑ "I feel like I can be more "myself" in India– people here are so pretentious sometimes, and everyone is trying to impress everyone else with what they have and where they work. I miss your smile." T, **USA**

❑ "You never cease to amaze me. All that you do or all that is done through you are assured of great success. As for me,

I spend much time studying in a master's of science program as I am trying to gain entrance into medical school. The classes and amount of information we are required to learn seems too much at times and also too boring! I have never really enjoyed the way medicine is practiced here – too impersonal, too much dependence on drugs and surgery, and often not very effective. I would comfort myself saying that if I became a doctor, I would practice differently." D **USA**

❏ "From Japan which was once called as one of the "Axis of Evil"! The other day I dreamt of you. You were like the hardest worker of an advancing company. With a mobile phone, much work, less sleeping, namely you seemed like a 1960s–70s Japanese hardest worker (though they didn't have a mobile phone). And I couldn't speak to you in that dream, because I felt it would be disturbing to you." S, **Japan**

❏ "In France, people think about the pleasure of food, the pleasure of sex, pleasure in work, pleasure with family, pleasure time. Always pleasure. (Not really a reality for all!). What do you think about this hedonism? Is that egoist for you? At work, people laugh about my vegetarianism. I laugh too! (Why not) And all the meal, there is some joke about this. Those people have a good heart. But they finally don't understand this choice, this feeling, and this difference. People like me, and maybe they don't respect me as I want. I have Faith in you too." N **France**

❏ "You are my teacher yes my fucking teacher because you teach me the more important things and it's incredible when you write to me is in the moment exactly when I more need your words. Believe me, Korak you are very important in the history of my life. Please Korak sorry for the distance I m have the last days. I m stay in Anantapur and don't eat meat fucking teacher I don't know the reason but I don't want to eat meat I have to give you thousands thanks because you put in my mind many important things. I love you fucking my brother one big kiss." M, **Spain**

❏ "I hope you remember me. I met one of the most extraordinary person in my life: you. Having the pleasure of seeing you at work made me stop and think. I really needed to do it. I'm so sorry I took so long before writing to you. I really have no excuse for that. But this time there's something important I have to tell you: I'm coming!!! I'll never forget you always smiling, gentle and at the same time so efficient. You made think about how small I am and made me want to be better. Every time I told my relatives and friends about my experience in India I've never forgotten to describe you. As you can understand the main reason why I coming back is to see you again and learn. My plane leaves from Italy on the 11th of April in the morning and arrives in Calcutta at 1:30 p.m. I'll be probably sleeping at the airport and reach you in the morning. I'll be back in Italy on the 30th. I couldn't afford more days." G. G **Italy**

Chapter 9

AN EXPERIMENT WITH MOTHER TERESA

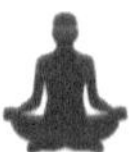

I came to Calcutta, now Kolkata to serve Humanity, around a year before Mother Teresa expired.

Unlike all the volunteers, I would never go to the Mother's House. There Mother Teresa lived, and people went to take her blessings or to see her. I was busy working in Nirmal Hirday, Kalighat serving the dying destitute, with my entire being. I was also going to the Howrah Station, the largest train station in Eastern India. I would go there early morning and scan all 23 platforms. Even the nearby under-passages, and the surrounding area.

I would search for any dying person and leprosy patients. Also look for people with maggots, unconscious or distressed women/children. Then would give them first aids or bring them to some hospitals or a Mother Teresa's charity home from there.

I was also teaching prostitute children and street children. This was at various charity schools in the Kalighat area of Calcutta. At the same time, I was also doing my Diploma course in Film Direction and Screenplay Writing in SRFTI. This is India's premiere Film School in Calcutta. So there were too much of management of time and energies.

I never went to Mother's Home to see Mother Teresa or even take her blessings. This was because I came to Calcutta to be in resonance with her spirit/soul. Also, for the works she did and not much to see her physical form.

It was a Black Saturday, the day after Good Friday. This day Jesus lay in the tomb after his death, according to the present version of the Christian Bible. Simon, a volunteer from England with a green stone ear dot in one ear, forced me. Took me to meet Mother Teresa during the evening Mass at the Mother House.

On the first floor chapel there, the Mass was going on. In the middle of the rectangular room, on the roadside was the altar. A moving image of Jesus Christ was there in a large cut-out. His skinny bone-protruding look, on the cross with a thorn crown and bleeding a lot.

In front of him are very fat, pink with health, white Priests. They wore bright red silk robes shouting with gold and luxury. Mother Teresa was sitting on a wheelchair right on the opposite wall and the most significant Sr. Luke stood behind her. She had a nickname of a 'bulldog.' She was Mother's ultimate and eternal bodyguard.

Diagonally, on Mother Teresa's right, at the top corner of the room, I was sitting with my simple working clothes. They were dirty after the whole day's work. I was studying the surroundings and the process of the Mass and also Mother and her body language.

As the Mass was continuing, I saw Mother looking at me/my side, and she smiles. I also saw that amongst the crowd of praying people from all over the world, there was a small path from me to Mother. No one was sitting on them, and it was clear.

I was already doing my Aatma Yoga meditations. I decided to take the most sacred step. I decided to leave my physical body behind and stand up with my spiritual body! I will teach this meditation to interested people when they qualify for it. You may contact me for this highest and most secret form of Satwik Aatma Yoga.

Anyway, I stood up and looked at my meditating body below. Then I looked at Mother praying with a row of beads and a stare, looking at her beloved Jesus. I walked up to Mother through that path amongst her devotees.

I stood in front of her looking at Jesus and in my back Mother sitting on her wheelchair. And I sat down.

I could feel the electricity running through my spine and the whole body, as I sat down on her lap and in her body. I looked at Jesus through her, then I looked at me sitting there in the corner, meditating. Looked up at Sr. Luke. I felt so many things in those few minutes.

Then I got up and went back to my physical body. I still have that feeling of electricity running through me since I felt it that day.

Chapter 10

KEY MILESTONES OF THE MEDIUM

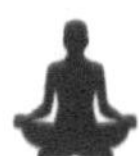

The Time-Line of Satwik Aacharay Korak Day and the works done 'through' him.

EARLY-LIFE: PARMATMA PRAPTI

Born on 1970 December 17th as Subhasish Sil in Agra, INDIA. The only son of a Para Jumping Instructor, in Indian Air Force. He studied in the Air Force School & Kendriya Vidhyalaya #1, Agra. He was the Head Boy, School-Captain. A National Champion in Inter-School level Singing and Drama. A topper in Secondary Level Exams at school-level in Hindi & English subjects. His favorite teachers were the AFS principal Ms. Sheela Jorge Russels, Ms. Kiran Basu and Mr. Moti Lal.

Later maneuvring his life, he studied until MSc. in Mathematics, at the Agra College. During those days, he also worked as a tutor, a salesman for Eureka Forbes and Fabers. At the age of 18, he received Aatma Yoga/Parmatma-Prapti Enlightenment. That would change his course of life. The ultimate mission for a human being, to be one with the Almighty, was revealed to him.

MILITARY LIFE: SATWIK RENUNCIATIONS

He earned the second position in the All-India Merit. That was the all-around exams for the best-educated Indian youth, the SSB. The Exam was at Varanasi, for getting selected in the Indian Military as an Officer. His Training was in INS Mandovi, Goa. In Cochin, Kerala he topped in the World Leadership Foundation Course. He secured the top three awards in the first three contests only, establishing a record there.

In 1996, precisely at the age of 25 1⁄2, he left the Military. That was to serve Humanity & Bharat, in reality. This he craved since his Aatma Yoga Enlightenment. He arrived in Calcutta. He had renounced his most favorite foods, material-thing and everyone he knew.

CALCUTTA: THE CHRISTIAN EXPERIENCE

He was Korak Day now, legally. He joined Mother Teresa's home for the dying-destitute. This was in Nirmal Hriday, Kalighat as an over-time volunteer. He also started learning Indian Classical Singing and Western Piano. Also studied about Films & Music theories in the USIS and NANDAN. Those days he also worked as a tutor and also joined Film Clubs. Korak lost 25 pounds in 5 months. Within a year he was selected in Satyajit Ray SRFTI. A film school for learning Film Direction & Screenplay Writing.

Soon he started going to the streets of Calcutta and Howrah Train Station. He helped the destitute there with the basics. He brought the dying-destitute, lepers, and maggot-filled helpless people to hospitals. He also volunteered at Brother Xavier's school for prostitute children. At a charity school for slum-children by Calcutta De Le'rue Al'Ecole and at the local L'Arshe Home. Korak called this experience his real Ph.D., and that ended in living with the slum-dwellers.

MY KARMA: AWARDED FILM

In 2001, friends from all over the world contributed to the film created 'through' Korak Day. That was KOLKATA'R KALI alias MY KARMA (was 8.9 on IMDb). Nicholas Stroebel, France; Shaun Ho, Taiwan; John Bowman, US; David Egan, Canada. Jorge Munita, Chile; Jatin Sarkar, India, and Dipak Patel, US were the contributors. Popular Indian Film-personalities like Moonmoon Sen, Arjun Chakraborty, Sabyasachi Chakraborty acted. National Award winners Anup Mukherji for Sound. Ashoke Bose for Art and Ashim Bose for Cinematography were part of the film.

Korak Day has vowed never to accept any Award. Never for his Parmatma-Prapti Works for Humanity and Bharat. Some of the crew told him that it was not just his film only. He sent this film to various film festivals. MY KARMA received 'Best Film' & 'Best Debut Director' Awards in 'New York Film Festival.' 'Best Screenplay' in Japanese 'Spiritual Film Festival' and a 'Grand Prix' in Poland. The film got a huge exposure, throughout the world, with 'Mother Teresa Film Festival.' Salute to the contributing friends, that such a unique film could reach humanity.

AAMAR NIJER MY OWN Inc.: DIPAK N PATEL

Few months before Mother Teresa died, Korak was taken to meet her on the Saturday of the Good Friday week. There he had an out-of-body experience with her that enriched his soul. Years later on the same day of Good Friday in 2002, Korak left volunteering at Missionary of Charity. This to start his own "Mission of Love," selfless-love as 'Aamar Nijer My Own.'

This was created to care for those people who were lonely, unloved, and friendless, either rich or poor. Very soon, Dr. Dipak N Patel from the USA joined as a contributing family member. Later his family too joined this Satwik Family,' just like Korak's blood- parents did earlier. Without his monthly sharing, in the 'Family Kitty,' all the work wouldn't have been possible. Humanity will always be indebted to his loving/caring heart!

SLUMS & VILLAGE WORK: ISLAM EXPERIENCE

The filth-filled and poverty-stricken Muslim slum named Butcher's Colony attracted his soul. So much that on 2002 July 2nd he started his work there. He was all alone, with no money. In a small room of the 'Torture Lane,' he started teaching little children and women. In-spite of the constraints, he vowed not to accept donations. That by projecting any human being with pity.

He started a 'Self-Developed Village Program.' That in that slum for helping the women to be financially independent.

Along with four schools in Narkeldanga, had branches in three villages outside Kolkata. All turned out to be Muslim villages too. Korak was too Humane to differentiate Humans by their external ideologies. He started a 'Satwik Ashram.' This for the old, mentally-unstable destitute women and the unwanted and needy children. In a very humble way, he has made over a hundred impoverished women his mother whom he calls DaDi. Meanwhile, he taught more than twelve thousand students in his 'Satwik Gurukuls.' Helped more than six hundred women & poor men, mostly Muslims, to get the dignity of a job.

SATWIK ART: SELFLESS LOVE

Korak created his first song 'Jiya Jae Na' during his SRFTI days, which became an instant hit. His Soul-stirring song 'Aami Manush' from his film 'My Karma' was a hit too. He continued making songs as 'Korak Gaan.' He has created 105 songs as a recording artist. They are mostly Mixed & Mastered in 'Sound City' or 'BR Films' Mumbai or Film Services, Kolkata. The songs are in three languages: Hindi, English, and Bangla.

He authored and Published 'When I Visited Earth,' 'Silent Symphony.' Also 'Kaamatur,' 'Songs of a Satwik Soul,' 'Kamokshsutra' and 'SSB Success Secrets.' Most books are available on Amazon and others online. In his Self-Dependent Villages, Korak created fashion with hand-woven Khadi-Silk. They had handcrafted embroidery & Zardozi works on them. He created apparel, saris, and other products and also produced countless 'hand-made and love-inspired' Feelings-Cards.

RENAISSANCE: SATWIK HUMANE

He spent six years of 'full-time' Christian experience. Then twelve years of 'full-time' Islamic experience. Post that, Korak Day decided to rejuvenate his working methods.

Chapter 11

SOUL DOST (FRIEND)

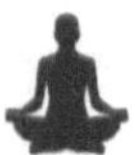

This is only the first book of the Aatma Yoga series. There will be many in the series revealing many Aatma Yoga aspects, practices, secrets. This will help humanity be in resonance with their own soul and be free from external prisons.

A Soul Dost is a 'Friend of your Soul.'

We all within us do not like many things that people do and also what we do, externally sometimes. But we still need to continue doing the things we dislike. This is due to various unavoidable circumstances. Thus we look for a person/place/group where we could just be ourselves. Also, be sure that we would be accepted and also that we will not lose them, ever. Like an Eternal Bonding! SoulDost provides you just that.

Here at SoulDost (through a website) we Satwik Friends and Satwiks are there for you. This is to share/care/ask/reply all your joys/sufferings/sadness/queries/happiness. As a caring Satwik friend/brother/sister/lover/mother/father etc.

There we will first know each other, share and do stuff together all towards the Aatma Yoga. Our objectives will be to help ourselves and others come out of our own problems ourselves.

It will be an Aatma Yoga Club. We will be serving/helping/ supporting/being there for each other's soul. Thus it will be non-external participation. You will be required to donate a Club Membership Fees in US$ as for a year, 5 years or for a Lifetime Memberships.

Then officially you have to fill up some Aatma Yoga Questionaire, and you will be given a Name. With that, you would start. No two members would know each other physically. This will be great fun and also of the most significant soul benefit for the participants. Know in more details by visiting our website souldost.com

Chapter 12

MITOCHONDRIA IMPLANTATIONS FOR YOU

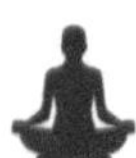

Here are some secrets that would make you win over any distraction. These will dilute your low morale and lead you towards a beautiful and worthy life:

★ "When you do good for others, they will, of course, do bad to you. But who cares, not you! A Satwik is doing all the good they could pay for their own Soul's good, for the Almighty, for humanity, for Earth and it's good. Not for those they are doing for, as they are actually a medium. So enjoy, keep doing good for others, more and more each day!"

★ "Life, which you are aware of, is one. Your happiness, contentment, and dream fulfillment will unlock by one key: be a Satwik."

★ "None of your relatives, friends, colleagues, no one will leave this world with you. Not even your bank balance, property, or celebrity status. The only thing that will come along post-death is those of your selfless good works."

★ "Replace depressions and feeling low/bad about something bad you have done. Put all your concentrations on doing good-actions for others, selflessly."

★ "A selfless work is that where you do that work without any expectations of the return of any kind, from that work."

★ "A human mother they say serves the child selflessly, which is mostly wrong. A human mother always expects returns from the child, and society would call that the duty of the child. Nothing wrong, but the word selfless is wrong to use here. Non-human mothers are actually selfless."

★ "When you get a bad thought to do something bad, then just know that someone is trying to lure you. Pay it back by doing two things good."

★ "If you can take care of a child not related to you in many ways, except humanity, then you are a selfless mother or father."

★ "Relationships get improved not by waiting upon them. But by tirelessly working upon them. And also by making relationships with your Soul: Aatma Yoga."

★ "Your body is a temple of the Almighty, and your mouth is the temple-door/window. Do not let any nonsense get inside it, so eat intelligently."

★ "You become what you eat. So do not eat a billionaire but be a spiritual billionaire. It needs luck and others to be a billionaire, but it's more rewarding to be a Soul Billionaire."

★ "Do not worry about anything in life, that will only bring the doctors closer and bank balance thinner. Do good things by becoming a Satwik, and all will be taken care of by the actual caretaker."

★ "Knowing your priorities in life and sticking to them is most important. This more important than taking breadth uselessly."

★ "Peace is permanent for you only when you accept that the peace you seek is impermanent."

★ "Slavery of any color or type is sin, listen to your heart. If you cannot listen to your heart being deaf, then come to me and become a Satwik, today."

★ "Keep rolling and be the role model."

★ "Joy becomes un-endable only when you know if you do not treat your soul well, it may just leave you, forever."

★ "Monetary satisfaction is a placebo, non-existent solution/ medicine. Imagine you received what you want monetarily. Soon a newer and higher monetary satisfaction number pops up. So, just enjoy life."

★ "Your unique brilliance within is non-existent until you work on its materialization. What are you waiting for, start now!"

★ "You are God just like me, but unless you work accordingly, you are just following the devil, within."

Chapter 13

HOW YOU COULD BE MILES AHEAD

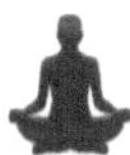

This is an optional chapter in this book. This chapter is for those who would like to take the next step from reading this book. If you feel to be a part of this soul-epoch and be/get a soul-dost (friend), then you are welcome to this chapter.

How you could take part

in our works and missions

for the benefit of humanity,

starting firstly, with yourself;

is the goal of this chapter.

Know Us

By the time you read this book, you would have known our missions, our work timeline since 1996 and also many testimonials.

Your Options

☐ Your <u>First Option</u> is to continue your life, precisely the way things were before this book. And if you have felt anything good within your soul, from this book, then our goal is fulfilled. We send you and your loved ones, pleasant wishes.

☐ The <u>Second Option</u> is Online. You could:

   i. ☐ **Thanks:** Send us a thank you note on our email address to the 'contributors' and the 'beneficiaries' of this book. Both of them are same: the endless dying destitute around the world, unwanted children, elderly and mentally unstable fellow humans whom no one wants anymore, the lonely/friendless/unloved people living anywhere between a palace and the streets. Korak Day is just a Satwik-Medium.

   ii. ☐ **U5to5:** If you want to and feel for our soul-epoch works, then you buy five more copies of the book and give them as a gift them to five people. Then you tell them to buy five more copies each and to give them to five more people, and so on. The royalties we will get from that will be a hard-earned fruit for the beneficiaries as mentioned earlier.

   iii. ☐ **BeSoulDost:** You could choose to be a soul (friend) dost by writing to us at korakdayfilms@gmail.com or directly through the website souldost.com You would be able to get a friend who would be interested in your soul and will be a soul friend forever, online. You would be able to share, care, and glare with the beauty of getting a SoulDost.

   iv. ☐ **Donate:** You could donate through our website or even directly to us in our bank for fulfilling our missions and for any of the followings: the endless dying destitute around the world, unwanted children, elderly and mentally unstable fellow humans whom no one wants anymore, the lonely/friendless/unloved people living anywhere between a palace and the streets.

   v. ☐ **Volunteer:** Be a Satwik Volunteer online. You could get more information through our website souldost.com. You could be anywhere on Earth and still, you could volunteer in the soul-epoch by just taking out an hour or more in a day and serve your soul and then for others. Responsibility and commitment will be your guiding light.

☐ The <u>Third Option</u> is by meeting the Satwik Aacharay Korak Day in Kolkata, INDIA (because we do not have branches in other cities/countries now). You could:

i. ☐ **Thanks:** Come visit us and thank the 'contributors' and the 'beneficiaries' of this book. Both of them are same: the endless dying destitute around the world, unwanted children, elderly and mentally unstable fellow humans whom no one wants anymore, the lonely/friendless/unloved people living anywhere between a palace and the streets. Korak Day is just a Satwik-Medium. Spend a few hours with our Humane-Family.

ii. ☐ **Volunteer:** Be a Satwik Volunteer in any of our present works according to your talent and wishes. You could get more information through our website souldost.com. Responsibility and commitment will be your guiding light. You could choose from 2 Days to 2 Years of various volunteering options, with or without stay/food and similarly with/without paying opportunities. Conditions applied.

iii. ☐ **Donate:** You could donate directly to our designated Satwik Manager. Or even straight to us in our bank for fulfilling our missions and for any of the followings: the endless dying destitute around the world, unwanted children, elderly and mentally unstable fellow humans whom no one wants anymore, the lonely/friendless/unloved people living anywhere between a palace and the streets.

iv. ☐ **BuildAlong:** We have projects running for building infrastructure and Satwik-Homes for our Humane-Family towards fulfilling our missions. Here you may Contribute/Donate/Buy according to the latest schemes available. You will get to know more details below and on the website.

v. ☐ **HomeStay:** This is an exciting option where you can stay in your Soul-Home in our branches, and we would be happy to be hospitable to you and your family. You could enjoy Satwik meals and an other-worldly environment. Here too you may Contribute/Donate/Buy according to the latest schemes available. You will get to know more details below and on the website.

vi. ☐ **ARTpatron:** This option is for those who are Art lovers and can appreciate and differentiate a piece of art from a product. We create films, music, books, etc. and you could Contribute/Donate/Buy according to the latest schemes available. You will get to know more details below and on the website.

Our Upcoming Projects

#1 ☐ **SOULdost HOMESTAY:** Be a part of Souldost-Homes [A HomeStay for you away from your own home, a Vanaprastha-Home for the affluent elderly, a Second Home as a permanent/temporary home for the rich-handicapped, a Conference Hall, a Picnic Spot, a Satwik Kitchen and a Satwik Family-Home for 50 elderly female Destitute]. We are constructing this project already, but due to lack of sufficient funds, it is taking a very long time. You could cheer this project up, with your generous contributions with/ without getting benefits as you would find below and also on our website.

Total Budget is $ 2 Million or Indian Rupee 12.5 Crore. You could either 'Donate Freely' or 'Get a Return Gift.' More details will be on our website. Meanwhile, if you want to donate freely, we are giving our bank details below.

The 'Get a Return Gift' option for this Project is:

#1 You Donate Rs. 60/$1 – Download a Certificate

#2 You Donate Rs. 1000/$15 – Download a Certificate + 05% Discount on Your HomeStays Rent + 05% on Food (02 days/year) Conditions Applied.

#3 You Donate Rs. 50,000/$750 – Certificate Sent to Your Mailing Address + 10% Discount on Your HomeStays Rent + 05% on Food (10 days/year) Conditions Applied.

#4 You Donate Rs. 2 Lakh/$2,900 – Certificate Sent to Your Mailing Address + 25% Discount on Your HomeStays Rent + 10% on Food (10 days/year) Conditions Applied.

#5 You Donate Rs. 5 Lakh/$7,250 – Certificate Sent to Your Mailing Address + 50% Discount on Your HomeStays Rent + 15% on Food (10 days/year) Conditions Applied.

#6 You Donate Rs. 20 Lakh/$28,900 – Certificate Sent to Your Mailing Address + 75% Discount on Your HomeStays Rent + 20% on Food (10 days/year) Conditions Applied.

#7 You Donate Rs. 50 Lakh/$72,200 – Certificate Sent to Your Mailing Address + 95% Discount on Your HomeStays Rent + 45% on Food (05 days/year) Conditions Applied.

#8 You Donate Rs. 75 Lakh/$108,300 – Certificate Sent to Your Mailing Address + 95% Discount on Your HomeStays Rent + 45% on Food (08 days/year) Conditions Applied.

#9 You Donate Rs. 1 Crore/$144,400 – Certificate Sent to Your Mailing Address + 95% Discount on Your HomeStays Rent + 45% on Food (12 days/year) Conditions Applied.

#10 You Donate Rs. 2 Crore/$288,800 – Certificate Sent to Your Mailing Address + 95% Discount on Your HomeStays Rent + 45% on Food (26 days/year) Conditions Applied.

#11 You Donate Rs. 7 Crore/$1,000,000 – Certificate Sent to Your Mailing Address + 95% Discount on Your HomeStays Rent + 45% on Food (80 days/year) Conditions Applied.

#2 ☐ **HARI DHAAM TEMPLE:** A Satwik & Secular Vishnu Temple with all his Avatars [a Satwik Hari Temple, a Gau–Shala for Indian-breed cows, a Ceremony Hall for festivals to enrich our souls, a Hari's Garden and a Family-Home for 50 elderly male Destitute & a Hari's Kitchen for delicious soul-satisfying foods. We are constructing this project already, but due to lack of sufficient funds, it is taking a very long time. You could cheer this project up, with your generous contributions with/without getting benefits as you would find below and also on our website.

Total Budget is $850,000 or Indian Rupee 5.5 Crore. You could either 'Donate Freely' or 'Get a Return Gift.' More details will be on our website. Meanwhile, if you want to donate freely, we are giving our bank details below.

The '<u>Get a Return Gift</u>' option for this Project is:

#1 You Donate Rs. 101/$2 – Download a Certificate.

#2 You Donate Rs. 1001/$15 – Certificate Sent to Your Mailing Address.

#3 You Donate Rs. 50,001/$750 – Certificate Sent to Your Mailing Address + Your Chosen Name + City/Town will be written on the back side brick of the Temple so that anyone going to that side can see. Conditions Applied.

#4 You Donate Rs. 2 Lakh/$2,900 – Certificate Sent to Your Mailing Address + Your Chosen Name + Full Address will be written on the side brick of the Temple so that anyone going to that side can see. Conditions Applied.

#5 You Donate Rs. 5 Lakh/$7,250 – Certificate Sent to Your Mailing Address + Your Chosen Name + City/Town will be written on a side pillar of the Temple so that anyone going to that side can see. Conditions Applied.

#6 You Donate Rs. 20 Lakh/$28,900 – Certificate Sent to Your Mailing Address + Your Chosen Name + Full Address will be written on a side pillar of the Temple so that anyone going to that side can see. Conditions Applied.

#7 You Donate Rs. 50 Lakh/$72,200 – Certificate Sent to Your Mailing Address + Your Chosen Name + City/Town will be written on the front pillar of the Temple so that everyone can see. Conditions Applied.

#8 You Donate Rs. 75 Lakh/$108,300 – Certificate Sent to Your Mailing Address + Your Chosen Name + Full Address will be written on the front pillar of the Temple so that everyone who enters can see. Conditions Applied.

#9 You Donate Rs. 1 Crore/$144,400 – Certificate Sent to Your Mailing Address + Your Chosen Name + City/Town will be prominently placed in the entrance of the Temple so that everyone who enters can see. Conditions Applied.

#10 You Donate Rs. 2 Crore/$288,800 – Certificate Sent to Your Mailing Address + Your Chosen Name + Full Address will be prominently placed in the entrance of the Temple so that everyone who enters can see. Conditions Applied.

#3 ☐ **ART PATRON** || Entertainment and Beyond inspired Films, Songs, Books created for Giving the elderly destitute and unwanted children a caring-family [3 feature Films, 15 Short Films, and 75 Music Videos]. We are creating arts in this project already, but due to lack of sufficient funds, it is taking a very long time. You could cheer this project up, with your generous contributions with/without getting benefits as you would find below and also on our website.

Total Budget is $4 Million or Indian Rupee 26 Crore. You could either 'Donate Freely' or 'Get a Return Gift.' More details will be on our website. Meanwhile, if you want to donate freely, we are giving our bank details below.

The 'Get a Return Gift' option for this Project is:

#1 You Donate Rs. 60/$1 – Download a Certificate

#2 You Donate Rs. 1000/$15 – Certificate Sent to Your Mailing Address + MORE (Many more benefits will come to you as this project becomes fulfilled, which you would be notified. Here you have to share on good faith, and you will receive well). Conditions Applied.

#3 You Donate Rs. 50,000/$750 – Certificate Sent to Your Mailing Address + Co-Producer Credit for one of our Feature Film + 0.03% Share of Profits + MORE (Many more benefits will come to you as this project becomes fulfilled, which you would be notified. Here you have to share on good faith, and you will receive well. The returns will be given until 20 years from the date of the film's release). Conditions Applied.

#4 You Donate Rs. 2 Lakh/$2,900 – Certificate Sent to Your Mailing Address + Co-Producer Credit for one of our Feature Film + 0.12% Share of Profits + MORE (Many more benefits will come to you as this project becomes fulfilled, which you would be notified. Here you have to share on good faith, and you will receive well. The returns will be given until 20 years from the date of the film's release). Conditions Applied.

#5 You Donate Rs. 5 Lakh/$7,250 – Certificate Sent to Your Mailing Address + Co-Producer Credit for one of our Feature Film + 0.30% Share of Profits + MORE (Many more benefits will come to you as this project becomes fulfilled, which you would be notified. Here you have to share on good faith, and you will receive well. The returns will be given until 20 years from the date of the film's release). Conditions Applied.

#6 You Donate Rs. 20 Lakh/$28,900 – Certificate Sent to Your Mailing Address + Co-Producer Credit for one of our Feature Film + 1.05% Share of Profits + MORE (Many more benefits will come to you as this project becomes fulfilled, which you would be notified. Here you have to share on good faith, and you will receive well. The returns will be given until 20 years from the date of the film's release). Conditions Applied.

#7 You Donate Rs. 50 Lakh/$72,200 – Certificate Sent to Your Mailing Address + Co-Producer Credit for one of our Feature Film + 2.25% Share of Profits + MORE (Many more benefits will come to you as this project becomes fulfilled, which you would be notified. Here you have to share on good faith, and you will receive well. The returns will be given until 20 years from the date of the film's release). Conditions Applied.

#8 You Donate Rs. 75 Lakh/$108,300 – Certificate Sent to Your Mailing Address + Co-Producer Credit for one of our Feature Film + 3.25% Share of Profits + MORE (Many more benefits will come to you as this project becomes fulfilled, which you would be notified. Here you have to share on good faith, and you will receive well. The returns will be given until 20 years from the date of the film's release). Conditions Applied.

#9 You Donate Rs. 1 Crore/$144,400 – Certificate Sent to Your Mailing Address + Co-Producer Credit for one of our Feature Film + 4.5% Share of Profits + MORE (Many more benefits will come to you as this project becomes fulfilled, which you would be notified. Here you have to share on good faith, and you will receive well. The returns will be given until 20 years from the date of the film's release). Conditions Applied.

#10 You Donate Rs. 2 Crore/$288,800 – Certificate Sent to Your Mailing Address + Co-Producer Credit for one of our Feature Film + 9% Share of Profits + MORE (Many more benefits will come to you as this project becomes fulfilled, which you would be notified. Here you have to share on good faith, and you will receive well. The returns will be given until 20 years from the date of the film's release). Conditions Applied.

#11 You Donate Rs. 7 Crore/$1,000,000 – Certificate Sent to Your Mailing Address + Co-Producer Credit for one of our Feature Film + 17% Share of Profits + MORE (Many more benefits will come to you as this project becomes fulfilled, which you would be notified. Here you have to share on good faith, and you will receive well. The returns will be given until 20 years from the date of the film's release). Conditions Applied.

#12 You Donate Rs. 18 Crore/$2,500,000 – Certificate Sent to Your Mailing Address + Co-Producer Credit for one of our Feature Film + 40% Share of Profits + MORE (Many more benefits will come to you as this project becomes fulfilled, which you would be notified. Here you have to share on good faith, and you will receive well. The returns will be given until 20 years from the date of the film's release). Conditions Applied.

Our Contact and Bank Details

Our contact address is:

Korak Day
c/o SATWIK HUMANE
3/3 Gauri Shankar Ghosal Lane,
Sastitala,
PO Narkeldanga
Kolkata 700011
INDIA
korakdayfilms@gmail.com

Bank Details for donations (we still do not have tax deduction benefits and the foreign currency accepting legal documents here yet, so you could use other options):

1. Name of Account: SATWIK HUMANE (for donors in India only)
   Name of Bank: Bandhan Bank
   Account Number: 10180006352326
   IFS Code: BDBL0001022
   Swift Code: BNDNINCC

2. Name of Account: KORAK DAY (for all currencies)
   Name of Bank: HDFC BANK
   Account Number: 50100167432320
   IFS Code: HDFC0001224
   Swift Code: HDFCINBBCAL

When you are donating money directly to Korak Day's account, it makes the transactions smooth and, when you mention that you are giving the money as a LOAN. Whatever way you Donate/Give/Contribute, all the funds will go for our missions of serving humanity, only:

If you are contributing to our ART Project as an ARTpatron, then you can give us directly to our Company's Bank Account as below.

3. Name of Account: SATWIK HUMANE
   Name of Bank: HDFC BANK
   Account Number: 50200032726640
   IFS Code: HDFC0001224
   Swift Code: HDFCINBBCAL

Also, you may send us a Cheque to "Korak Day" or Western Union Money Transfer in the same name.

EPILOGUE

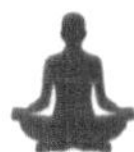

Life is beautiful only for those who open the doors within. Then only they can decode the secrets they have, all of us have, within ourselves.

The present-day world and its system would not allow such ideas to flourish. Not in the slavery-driven world, we have these days. I can say this because I know what I had to do/go through following this path to Aatma yoga since 1996 August 16th.

Coming this far was difficult, but following which path is easy? It's hard work in every track. Some people get things overnight due to their good luck or suitable coincidence. But still, for them too, it's a considerable task/work, to maintain that success.

I have mentioned earlier that there is an important secret for a person who wants to be successful in life. She/he has to accept all the failures and struggles that come along. It's not the failure of getting suitable results, but the success of trying successfully by not giving up.

Come, let us build a lasting relationship. I welcome you to our website souldost.com and also at korakdayfilms@gmail and help me, in whatever way you want to. Come let's make things the best, for us and for the entire humanity and nature.

This book is just introducing Aatma Yoga to you. Practicing the higher Aatma Yoga would be the next step with a Satwik Aacharay. You are welcome to our Satwik Ashram in Kolkata, INDIA.

Other Books of KORAK DAY

SSB SUCCESS SECRETS
(Amazon #1 Bestseller)

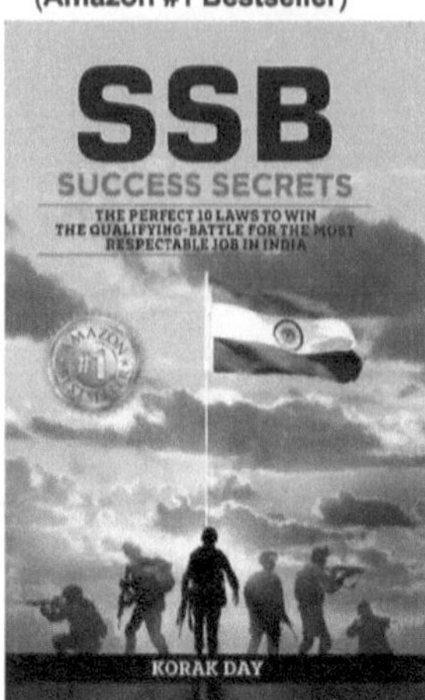

KAAMATUR

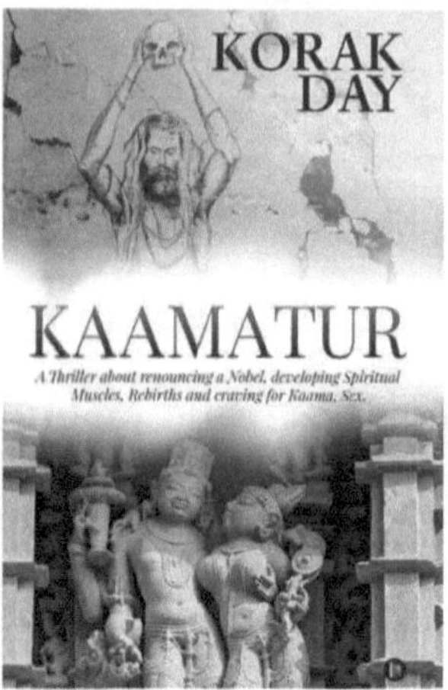

WHEN I VISITED EARTH

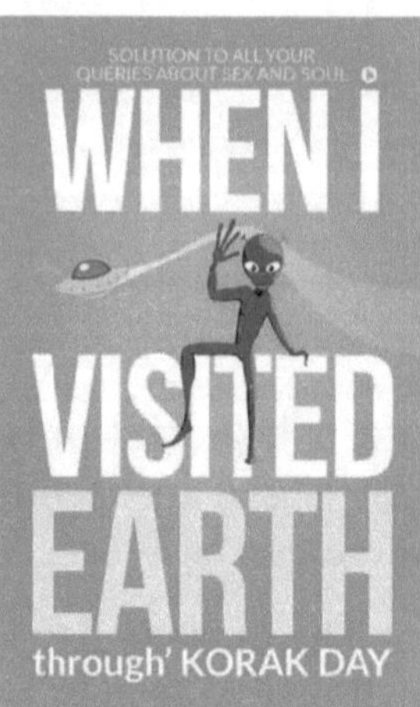

SONGS OF A SATWIK SOUL
(A Book of Poetries)

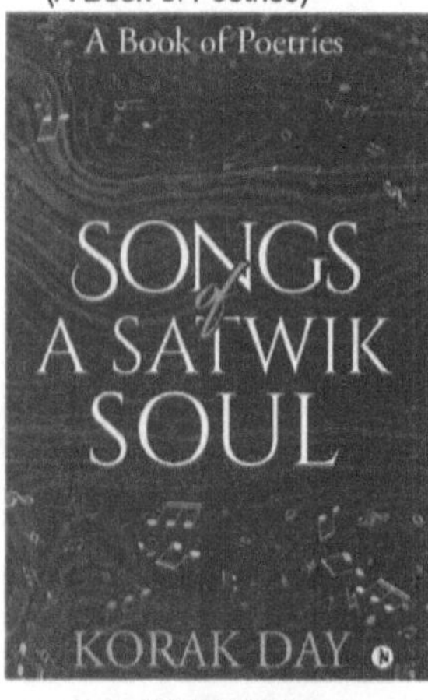

KAMOKSHSUTRA

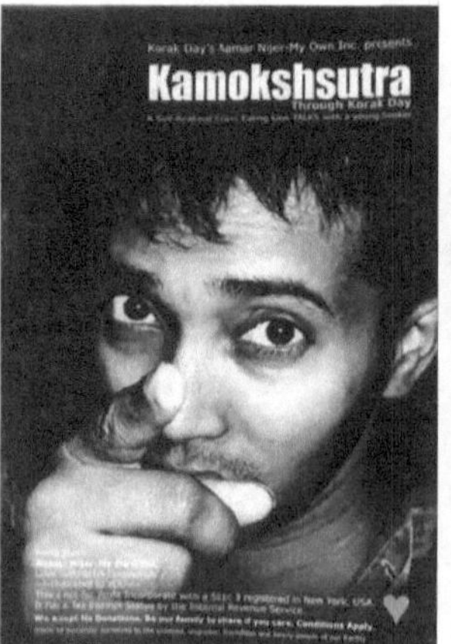

THE SILENT SYMPHONY

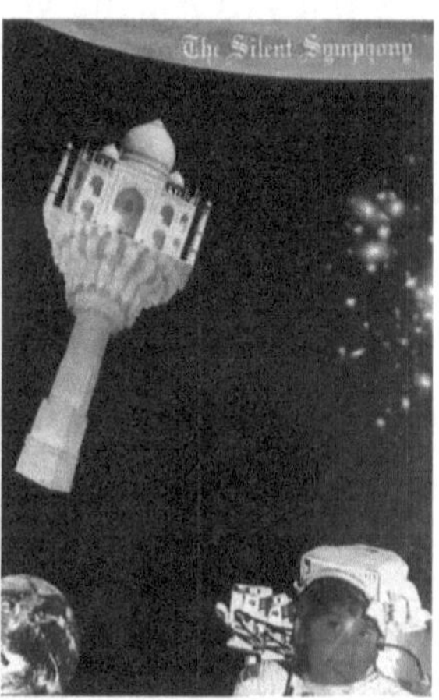

SEX YOGA

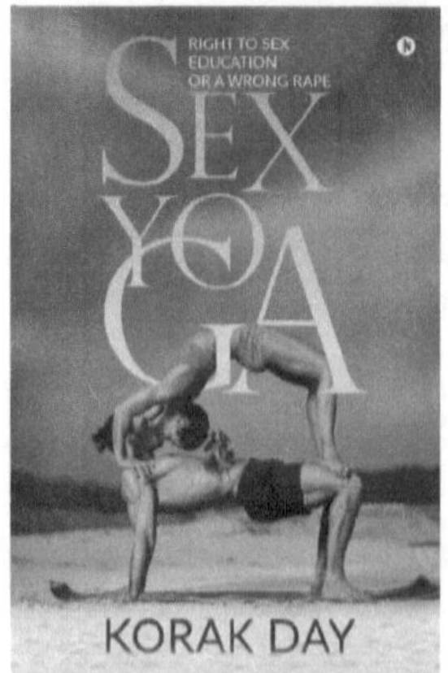

www.ingramcontent.com/pod-product-compliance
Lightning Source LLC
Chambersburg PA
CBHW031144250726

48655CB00002B/824